RICHARD HITTLEMAN

You've seen him on TV.
Perhaps you've read one of his five original Bantam books.
Now, in one great volume, the man who has introduced the practice of Yoga to more people throughout the world than any living authority adds an essential dimension to the Yoga science, affording layman, student and teacher the chance to become aware of every important method of Yoga, to grasp the ancient secrets and to take the 8 wondrous steps to health and peace . . .

Bantam Books by Richard Hittleman
Ask your bookseller for the books you have missed

RICHARD HITTLEMAN'S GUIDE TO YOGA MEDITATION
RICHARD HITTLEMAN'S INTRODUCTION TO YOGA
WEIGHT CONTROL THROUGH YOGA
YOGA: THE 8 STEPS TO HEALTH AND PEACE
YOGA NATURAL FOODS COOKBOOK
YOGA 28 DAY EXERCISE PLAN

YOGA:
THE 8 STEPS TO
HEALTH AND PEACE

RICHARD HITTLEMAN

*This low-priced Bantam Book
has been completely reset in a type face
designed for easy reading, and was printed
from new plates. It contains the complete
text of the original hard-cover edition.*
NOT ONE WORD HAS BEEN OMITTED.

RLI: $\dfrac{\text{VLM 11 (VLR 9-12)}}{\text{IL 10-adult}}$

YOGA: THE 8 STEPS TO HEALTH AND PEACE
A Bantam Book

PRINTING HISTORY
Deerfield Communications Corporation edition | 1975
Bantam edition | October 1976

All rights reserved.
Copyright © 1975 by Richard L. Hittleman.
*This book may not be reproduced in whole or in part, by
mimeograph or any other means, without permission.
For information address: Bantam Books, Inc.*

ISBN 0-553-02116-8

Published simultaneously in the United States and Canada

*Bantam Books are published by Bantam Books, Inc. Its trade-
mark, consisting of the words "Bantam Books" and the
portrayal of a bantam, is registered in the United States
Patent Office and in other countries. Marca Registrada. Bantam
Books, Inc., 666 Fifth Avenue, New York, New York 10019.*

PRINTED IN THE UNITED STATES OF AMERICA

0 9 8 7 6 5 4 3 2 1

CONTENTS

To SELF—
that desires and requires nothing,
but to which, nonetheless, all things are
knowingly or unknowingly dedicated.

CREDITS

Photographs—Al Weber
Illustrations—Lorenzo André
Models for the Photographs:
Patricia Cederwall
Margie Monroe
Charles Muir
Les Fulgham

PART I

The Great Conspiracy

*We see ourselves as that which
we are not—and that which we
are we fail to recognize.*

—Richard L. Hittleman

Chapter 1

Desire-Action:
The Illusion of Fulfillment

It has always seemed to me that the most astonishing information that can be conveyed to a human being in this life is that the fulfillment of all his hopes and desires lies within himself, *and only within himself!* Although understanding this, a person has comprehended all the truth there is, and although this truth can be stated as I have above—in the most simple and direct manner—the very large majority of people is prone to dismiss this extraordinary pronouncement almost immediately upon hearing or reading it. And even among those who may recognize that there is something of the greatest significance in a statement such as, "The kingdom of heaven lies within," most find that a peculiar forgetfulness of this significance occurs and that long periods of time can elapse before they give it the attention it warrants. In short, the majority of mankind reacts to the startling precept: "You will find what you are seeking only within yourself" as though it had little, if any, relevance to mankind.

What a remarkable situation! Throughout his lifetime a man strives with all of his being, engaging in a never-ending series of the most trying, exasperating, tedious, and frequently outlandish activities in the hope of realizing at least partial happiness, peace, and fulfillment —objectives in which he is continually frustrated—and yet, when he is informed that this realization lies closer to him than his eyes or his heart he generally disregards such information, or is inclined to forget it within a matter of moments! If the media were to promote the idea that fulfillment in life could be achieved by journeying to some remote region of the Arctic, think of the multitude who would clog the routes, readily enduring whatever hardships and dangers are inherent in such a journey. And yet, although numerous highly "reliable sources" have, since time immemorial, pointed to that place where all of men's problems are resolved without taking a single step and without the frantic, often absurd strivings in which they are continually involved, such incredible information falls upon the deaf ears of a very high percentage of those to whom it is conveyed.

Two men sit side by side and are instructed by a Master. "To find peace," he states, "look within and find your Self." The first man, in a way that we shall understand later, has an immediate realization of the significance of this instruction. He undertakes to reflect upon and apply, in certain prescribed procedures, what he has been told. In due course this practice results in his enlightenment and subsequent liberation. He becomes free from suffering and is at peace. For the second man this instruction has no real meaning. He hears the identical words as the first man but is unable to comprehend them because they pertain to a dimension of existence with which he has no conscious contact. His rational, reasoning mind (to which he submits all data) has no frame of reference for the illogical input. It cannot conceive of where "within" is to be located, or how it shall find a "self" other than the one that it believes it knows perfectly well. Consequently, perhaps immediately, perhaps after some little consideration, the words of the Master are dismissed as irrelevant. It is in this sense that the second man is "deaf," that he does not have "ears to hear." Spiritual knowledge, eso-teric doctrines, metaphysical principles, occult "secrets" can all be revealed in his presence; to him they are meaningless, even nonsensical because he has no direct awareness of that dimension whence they originate and to which they pertain. So although this man's existence in what he knows as the "world" is, in actuality, totally sustained through another dimension (the "within") this other dimension remains strangely obscured, hidden from him. The great riddle therefore becomes, "How is it that a man can be ignorant of that which is the source of his life and be unaware of the one and only *reality* of his existence: the Self?

This riddle has formed the nucleus from which the most profound schools of oriental philosophy have evolved. In these philosophies one frequently encoun-ters the Sanskrit term *maya,* a fascinating word that is used to describe that state of consciousness in which the "deaf" man functions. It is a state of illusion and forgetfulness, a type of hypnosis. That is, a man, for-getting his true nature, his real identity, forgetting *who he is,* identifies himself with a body and a mind and attaches himself to the objects and conditions that his mind interprets as the "world." He then attempts to possess, manipulate, and function among these objects and conditions in a way that he believes will result in his happiness and fulfillment. This assumption consti-tutes man's "fall" and is responsible for all of his sub-sequent difficulties, which in oriental philosophies are described as "sufferings."

To put it another way: in the state of maya, I am fully convinced that my body, and elements that I refer to as "my mind," comprise my "self." (I may also admit to a "soul" but even if I regard myself as "religious" this is the vaguest of intangibles and plays a meaning-ful part in my life, if at all, on only the rarest occa-sions.) Once the image of the "self," the "I," the "ego" is firmly established in my consciousness, I am indeed an "individual." I see and feel my self as being differ-ent, separate, apart from all of the other selves that surround me. I now find my self to be comprised of a body, senses, emotions, and a mind and these quickly infuse in me the concept of "threat." That is, they advise me that my self is subject to a very broad spectrum of undesirable experiences ranging from minor discomforts to total extinction. As a consequence I am made to understand that the business of my life will be not only to protect my self from whatever may threaten it physically, but from everything that would diminish any aspect of it and make it appear as less than it wishes to be; it demands protection from every type of mental and emotional pain and adversity. Simultaneously, I must increase my self, build it, develop it, inflate it, aggrandize it, make it real and permanent and provide it with security in all situations. Once accepting this I can no longer distinguish between the true, real, nonfragmented Self of my original state and those attributes of body, mind, senses, and emotions which comprise my self. I identify totally with the latter and the Self becomes "myself." Now I exist in the state of maya. Here, I have no conscious knowledge of the progression of events—of the "fall"—described in the preceding paragraphs. Now, nothing is of greater importance than myself (no matter how altruistic the role in which it is cast). I become wholly immersed in mayic activities. Seeking the protection and aggrandizement of myself, I contrive endlessly to experience success without failure, pleasure without pain, happiness without despair, love without complications. I engage in those activities which my reasoning, rational, logical mind, and my emotions and senses, have informed me will accomplish these ends. In my state of maya I fail to understand that the selves I see all about me are also in this state of illusion and that the activities with which they are involved, those which *their* senses, emotions, and reasoning minds have directed them to engage in, cannot lead to the realization of the desired goals any more than can my own.

The fact that I and those around me never seem to achieve our objectives in the ultimate sense, that we find human dissatisfaction and unrest wherever we turn, does not shake our collective confidence that we are nonetheless on the right path. That is, the fact that whatever fulfillment we appear to experience is inevitably followed by the need for additional fulfillment, or that the peace we gain is soon disturbed by one or another event, we attribute to the inadequacy of our actions. We continue to convince one another through the "Emperor's New Clothes" syndrome, through the most remarkable universal conspiracy, that sooner or later, individually or collectively, we *shall* hit upon the correct pattern of actions and our objectives *will* be achieved.

And so we press on: we will endeavor to impose peace upon the world, sweep out the old guard, get the poor off welfare, run the hippies out of town, nationalize the oil industry, attend the proper group therapy sessions, fall in love with the right person, raise a family, travel to exotic lands, get that job promotion, drop out and join the movement to legalize marijuana, buy a sleek foreign car, and discover the ultimate deodorant; then we shall surely, at last, be fulfilled. Let us therefore dismiss our aeons of previous failures and pursue the *right* course of action which will, *this time*, bring about the desired ends.

The continuing call of my fellow conspirators is for *action*. I agree. I fully accept the proposition that "action is necessary to satisfy desire," and I learn that particular actions are necessary to satisfy particular desires. I may, on occasion, examine the *type* of desire and the *type* of action but *I never question the validity of desire and action themselves.*

If I read that, in a serious discussion of man's activities, no value distinction is made between a questionable enterprise such as the "search for the ultimate deodorant," and a highly noble endeavor as "the cultivation of world peace," I may grow indignant. There is a most crucial point to be made here: my indignation is an overt reaction of my self, the ego. It righteously asserts that some activities are inherently more meritorious than others. The collective ego of the conspirators advances this concept in the guise of promoting human dignity and conscience; by so doing it lends validity to a value scale of activities. This is the very trap that ensnares the self in the belief that action can result in fulfillment and that different types of action result in different types of fulfillment. The startling truth is that *no activity is more meaningful than another in effecting my true fulfillment, no matter how sincere the resolve, no matter how ardent the pursuit, no matter how apparent the success in bringing it to a satisfactory conclusion, no matter how frequent the change from one mode of action to another!*

I have no difficulty in understanding this as it pertains to certain basic *physical* desire-action patterns. If I am thirsty, I drink; if I am tired, I sleep. Neither is more important than the other and although each of these desires has been fully satisfied I certainly do not equate this satisfaction with permanent fulfillment. I know that I shall soon thirst and tire again but in the meantime, having temporarily satisfied these basic desires, I can get on with the real business of life—of satisfying my more important, more significant desires. So, although I know without doubt that I shall thirst and drink, tire and sleep throughout my lifetime, my perspective in the state of maya is circumscribed to the extent that I seem incapable of applying this vital knowledge to what I have conceived of as the "really important" business of my life. I fail to apprehend the process of *continually alternating opposites*: there is a never-ending cycle of pleasure and pain, happiness and despair, success and failure. The time will never come when I have finally, through my persistence, hard work, ingenuity, and good luck beaten the game. In my hypnotic condition I accept the party line and learn to conceive of pleasure apart from pain, happiness apart from despair, and success apart from failure. I then contrive, with every resource at my command, to experience one without the other, to, in the words of the popular song, "accentuate the positive" and "eliminate the negative." What a hopeless endeavor!

I do not discern that pleasure and pain are inherent in one another, that they are two ends of the same stick, that I cannot hold one without simultaneously holding the other. If I strive to achieve happiness I shall certainly experience a corresponding degree of misery, for one is as certain to evolve from the other as day turns into night. In the state of maya I am continually diverted by my fellow conspirators (and my own "rational" mind) from confronting the truth that would transform my existence: pleasure and pain are one, success will certainly alternate with failure, it is

6

only a question of time until my present, hard-won peace of mind degenerates into new turmoil, forcing me into a whole further series of activities in an attempt to regain tranquillity. Once this fundamental Law of Continually Alternating Opposites penetrated my consciousness I would perceive that it covers the entire range of human endeavors and that failure to quench my thirst for permanent security, permanent peace, permanent fulfillment is due not to my inadequate or incorrect action, but is the result of my belief that action, as I know it, can culminate in anything that is permanent and fulfilling!

In questioning the value of action—mind you, not the *type* of activities in which I am involved and whether they are noble or base, *but the whole conception of action itself*—I would be led to examine the phenomenon of *desire,* for I would discover, quite naturally, that it is desire that engenders action. Put in the most simple possible terms the pattern is this: I *want* such-and-such, and therefore I must *do* such-and-such to have it. This is so basic, so axiomatic, that our life can generally be described entirely in terms of the desire-action pattern. I am taught to determine on a minute-to-minute as well as on a lifelong basis what it is I need and want, and to implement the actions that will satisfy these desires. This process has become so "natural" that, without rebellion, I accept (I even encourage) the experience of a never-ending series of desires that must be translated into a never-ending series of corresponding actions. After all, if some or most of my desires are not satisfied, there is hardly a single fellow conspirator who is not delighted to provide me with an almost infinite number of alternative courses of action or suggest how I may exchange my impossible, fantasy desires for more realistic ones.

However, if, as stated above, the futility of the actions with which I have been continually involved were to become apparent to me (through my understanding of the Law of Continually Alternating Opposites), and this led to an examination of *desire*—again, not the relative merit of one desire as opposed to another, *but the whole conception of desire itself*—I would indeed open a Pandora's box. I would be forced to reflect upon the nature of desires. Where do they come from? Why do they endlessly succeed one another? Why, when I appear to have satisfied a long-standing desire of major consequence, is my sense of fulfillment so short-lived? Are desires, as I have always believed, "natural"? What if I am never able to satisfy my strongest desires?

This line of questioning, if pursued in depth, would cast desire in a completely different and extremely significant light. I would have to reevaluate the role that desire plays in my existence, and I would gain an insight into the desire-action relationship that could lead to a highly disturbing conclusion: desire engenders action, but the action that I undertake to satisfy the desire not only frequently necessitates a whole group of attendant actions, but tends to generate a multitude of new desires! This cycle, which, in the innermost depths of my being I would detect is responsible for a continual frustration, a ground base of suffering, is obviously an eternal one. That is, if desires (which arise from an unknown source and which I seem helpless to prevent) require actions that ultimately prove fruitless in providing the permanent peace, security, and fulfillment that I seek, and if my very involvement in these actions can generate a series of new desires for which I must undertake a corresponding series of new actions, at what point will this process terminate? When and where shall I cease to suffer and, at last, find peace? My reasoning, rational, logical mind can only respond with "Never." And if my self were able to view the situation from an even more profound vantage point, it would add, "Not in death, which is but an extension of life, and not in an infinite number of succeeding lifetimes and deathtimes." This cycle is eternal.

(Desires, and the still-to-manifest effects of their corresponding actions [karma] do not evaporate into nothingness at the time of death. The physical body dissolves but desires are unfinished business; they remain in a subtle seed form awaiting another vehicle for subsequent expression and potential fulfillment. As with all desire, action eventually ensues. Here, action results in what is known as "reincarnation": a new body provides the needed vehicle. *It is the desire that incarnates;* the body is born into the physical world with the seed of previous desires contained therein. [What do you mean, "I didn't ask to be born"? Of course you did.] Because desires are infinite and thus cannot be satisfied during any lifetime of a physical body, the lifetimes themselves become infinite! And even when the universe is withdrawn and temporarily sleeps, that is, when it is in its "night," its *potential* rather than *manifest* state, the seeds of desire of the individual selves remain with it, also sleeping, also potential. When an astronomical period of time has elapsed and the universe once again manifests on all of its planes, when it is once again in its "day" period, the desire seeds manifest with it and each individual self takes on another endless series of bodies to nurture these seeds. This day-night cycle of creation is, likewise, eternal.)

But the resourcefulness of my fellow selves in maintaining the desire-action-fullfillment illusion, in diverting me from examining too closely the hat from which the rabbit is pulled, is dazzling. If, from time to time, I voice my fleeting suspicion that we may be collective victims of some stupendous self "put-on"; if, in a moment of particularly intense frustration or anguish I am led to question the basic fabric of the mayic plane, I find that the selves around me are instantly transformed into miraculous combinations of magicians-therapists. What cunning, what tenacity, what sleight of hand they display! At one or another such time I may be advised, either directly or through implication:

- Everyone has difficult periods; these things have a way of straightening themselves out; time heals all wounds; things will look better next week.

- Have another martini (or another joint).

- Find yourself a good analyst; discover what your "hang-ups" are, how to better relate to people, how to get it all together, how to function as a meaningful member of society.

- See your clergyman; confess your sins, rid yourself of guilt, become a more spiritual person.

- Your sex life is inadequate; you need an exciting romance.

- "Think positively." This makes you dynamic, forceful, optimistic, successful.

- Psychodrama helps work out hostility and depression.

- Why don't you go back to college?

- With a hairpiece, a new wardrobe, and the loss of twenty-five pounds your self-image will really be enhanced. You'll be beautiful, desirable, glamorous, the envy of your friends, the life of every party.

- A better job will provide more security.

- You need a purpose in life; learn to give of yourself and help people; become involved in a meaningful crusade and it will all seem worthwhile.

- Love conquers all. You must learn how to love.

- Have you tried vitamin E? Astrology? Golf? Exorcism? Folk dancing? ESP? Filmmaking? You may have natural abilities, hidden talents that you've never explored.

How can I contest such wisdom? I am overwhelmed. The principle is very clearly conveyed to me: if I begin to suspect that the emperor is not really wearing any clothes at all I must be hallucinating; if I entertain the notion that it is the inmates who are running the asylum I am under some severe stress. Fortunately there are things I can do to cure my afflictions. The above list represents only a small number of possibilities. I am once again persuaded, as I have been persuaded for as many times as there are "grains of sand on the banks of the Ganges," that I simply have yet to find that proper course of action which will yield fulfillment. My faith renewed, my immobilization passed, I rejoin the conspiracy. I forge forward in quest of new horizons. The bluebird of happiness may be lying in wait just beyond any one of them.

Chapter 2

Ordinary Mind:
Keeper of the Keys

In chapter 1 we described a "fall" or transformation from the original state of SELF to the *mayic* condition of my self. In the latter I think of this self as being comprised of elements that include (1) a body with senses; (2) a mind with which emotions are somehow associated and that can abstract such things as a "soul" and a "conscience." When I speak or think of "myself" I have reference to all of these, but upon close observation I detect that I do not consider the *essence* of my self to be equally present in all. For example, I view this essence as being in my *body* in only a limited way. I do not minimize the importance of my body but I am consciously aware of this body in two fundamental ways: as it makes known its needs, and as it is fitted to appear in the arena. Its needs are widely diverse and range from the desirability of having its teeth brushed to the act of procreation. The greater majority of these needs are, as time passes, met semiautomatically, frequently almost unconsciously. Even in gratifying those

11

which are of a more compelling or even sensual nature
—such as hunger or the sexual urge—my mind can be
preoccupied. Evidently, then, I am able to meet my
physical needs with minimal involvement of the self
and I am left with the impression that only a modicum
of my self is localized in my body and senses. Pain or
discomfort can require my more continuous attention
but this does not alter my notion that the essence of
my self is only partially in my body.

I can become deeply involved in grooming my body
—in adorning and shaping it to fulfill a manufactured
image. And because this image continually changes I
can devote the better part of my entire life to such
efforts, as do a great number of my fellow conspirators. In this case I am very much aware of my body
since it becomes the paramount consideration of my
existence. But the fruits of these efforts, whatever they
may be, *are not realized by my body.* A romantic con-
quest, winning a sports event, acclaim for an artistic
performance, compliments on my latest wardrobe or
suntan provide small physical enjoyment, for although
the body is the vehicle for such victories the satisfaction is cerebral and emotional. *It is my mind, and my
emotions, that savor the triumphs.* My body is simply
in the arena. It is entered in events as a trainer enters
his horse in various shows. The successes or failures
that result from these events are experienced primarily
by the trainer (mind), seldom by the horse (body). I
can now understand that I really view my mind-body
relationship in a peculiar manner: my mind is the
repository of intelligence; attached to it is a creature,
an animal, a body that transports my mind and that my
mind directs. Mind steers this body on numerous
courses from which it hopes to derive varying degrees
of pleasure and fulfillment. (If, because of some physical deformity or other negative condition, or through
the teachings of certain religions or philosophies, I become ambivalent to my body, I live all the more in my
mind.)

So it is that when I reflect on the concept of my
"self" as it relates to my body, I perceive (1) that my
physical needs can more frequently than not be satisfied
almost unconsciously with what is apparently minimal

"self" involvement; (2) that those events in which my body plays the major role are, nonetheless, experienced primarily by my mind (and emotions). My analysis therefore discloses that I identify the greater part of my "self" with my mind, that I *live principally in my mind, not in my body.*

I can well understand how this situation has developed: although I do appreciate the marvel of my physical organism I am also acutely cognizant of its limitations. But my mind!—what an incredible and *unlimited* instrument we have here. I can lose parts of my body, certain of its processes can be impaired and it can even become immobile, but my mind will continue to function. Through mind all things are possible. Whatever I seek to know and understand can be forthcoming from my mind. Utilizing those qualities ascribed to it—reason and logic—and with its ability to perceive, discriminate, interpret, and evaluate, it performs for me a multitude of indispensable and miraculous functions. Small wonder that I and my fellow conspirators worship our individual and collective mind and are forever informing one another of its astounding accomplishments and infinite possibilities. "The mind of man!" we proclaim. "What is beyond its capabilities?"

My reverence for mind is due, in no small part, not only to how it directs my body but to the service it performs with respect to desire-action-fulfillment. When my mind apprehends my desires it evaluates them and advises me of the actions required for their fulfillment. And it has the ability to continually alter or modify its counsel in any degree necessary to aid me in dealing with changing situations and changing desires. Faithful and wondrous servant! If it errs, if it fails to provide me with a satisfactory solution to a particular problem or with what I regard as a fulfilling conclusion in a given situation, I am quick to forgive it. I recognize the numerous extenuating circumstances that are involved. It can hardly be held responsible for bad luck, unforeseen occurrences, or incomplete input. And immediately upon the heels of any ineptitude it is able to revise, rectify, reevaluate; additionally, it is eternally ready to be "improved" and "expanded." What more could one ask? No, despite what I interpret as an "occasional failure" I feel completely justified in placing unqualified reliance upon my mind to cope with all circumstances in which I find myself; it is inconceivable that it would serve in any capacity other than that which is ultimately in my best interests. After all, it is *my* mind, an indispensable part of *me*. It is at once my adviser, my friend, my confidant. I even spend many hours each day engaged in silent conversation with it and I grow extremely uncomfortable when I imagine myself in a situation where its full faculties would not be available. The thought of mental disorders and abnormalities fills me with apprehension. How could I function without my mind? What would become of me? My existence without a fully operating mind is frightful to contemplate. All of these impressions contribute to my conviction that, with several relatively insignificant exceptions, my mind is omnipotent. I grant it executive privilege; it can do little wrong; there is no need to question its allegiance to me or my dependence upon it.

This view that we hold of our minds, this dependent way in which we relate to them, this essence of "self" with which we invest them is established early in life and is reinforced on an almost second-to-second basis through the years. Early on, we accept mind and the way it appears to function in maintaining and fulfilling our lives as naturally as we accept our heartbeat. The necessity of questioning this acceptance is so remote that it has long since ceased to occupy our consciousness. But now we *are* going to question our mind acceptance and it is urgent that the reader become consciously aware of the extent to which he has been an unaware participant in this acceptance. It would, therefore, be highly meaningful for the reader to spend several minutes at this point in examining how he regards and relates to his mind. If he will do that *now* and refer to the above commentary as background material he will probably conclude that this commentary expresses, quite accurately, the situation that obtains. This would be a revelation of paramount importance. . . .

Our fellow conspirators encourage us, in the name of furthering the glorification of mind, to investigate the magnificence of its functions and explore its limitless potential. In so doing we are gainfully occupied and effectively diverted, for in the uncovering of endless wonders, amid the splendors of a new virus and increasingly remote galaxies, who would commit the sacrilege of questioning the homage paid to this miraculous "mind of man"? To seriously undertake such an investigation would be to invite the greatest concern of our fellow mind worshipers, for they would perceive in this a threat of the first magnitude. The unquestioning trust that is placed in the ability of mind to ultimately interpret the most perplexing phenomena of the universe as well as to provide efficacious guidance in all situations is one of the principal pillars of the mayic structure and must stand firm at any cost. Consequently, any prospective defector, suspected of chipping away—however lightly—at these pillars will feel the full weight of the conspiracy upon him. Ridicule, scorn, and even enforced "therapy" are but a few of the techniques utilized. Usually these are successful in discouraging the investigator; only one who has experienced a profound "awakening" will persist. (Without going into details, mention to those at the college you attend or at your favorite bar that you are questioning the ability of mind to offer valid guidance in the quest for fulfillment and note the generally disdainful reaction. Persist in this over a period of time and note the increasing hostility toward you of your companions.) But proceeding under the premise that the reader may have been led to peruse this book because he *has* experienced an awakening we will now incur the wrath of the mayic agents by pursuing exactly such an investigation. And just as under a special type of examination the concept of fulfillment-through-action was revealed to be an illusion, responsible for continual frustration and suffering, so by subjecting our worship of mind and our identification of self with mind to scrutiny from what we shall term an "extra-mayic perspective" we shall find that the those truths which emerge reveal to us that the mind is equally the perpetrator of our bondage.

In my everyday life I use the word "mind" to designate what I regard as a repository of certain essential components of my "self," among which is a "brain." I have no perception, no subjective or objective evidence whatsoever of a "mind" but I do have objective evidence of a "brain" and I frequently use these two words interchangeably. Almost always when I speak of my "mind" I am actually referring to my brain, to my computer. Although the word "computer" is relatively new in our common vocabulary the brain has always functioned as a computer. The highly sophisticated computers currently in operation were, of course, devised by the brain and reflect but the tiniest fraction of its abilities. The brain is every bit as incredible as I have always believed. Indeed, it is so incredible that I fail to notice the power it has appropriated in the guise of "serving" me.

A familiar theme in science fiction is that of the computer "taking over." The brain takeover that *has actually transpired within each individual in the mayic state* is the prototype of this plot. Having been devised to serve in the capacity of a servant, the brain has become the master. In its takeover it has been abetted by cohorts—other elements that we attribute to mind. As we examine the phenomenon of this takeover it is necessary that we make a very clear distinction between the mind that we conceive of as the brain, together with attendant components, and Supreme Intelligence or Universal Mind. We shall, therefore, apply the prefix "ordinary" to the former and designate it as *"ordinary mind."*

When I concluded that my self is more in my mind than in my body I did, indeed, arrive at the correct conclusion, but I am correct in a way that is much different than I would have theorized. I discover that ordinary mind does a most remarkable thing: *it manufactures and maintains the illusion of a "self."* This illusionary self (that is referred to as "I," "me," "myself") obscures my Real SELF, my True "I" as it exists in my original, pure, spotless, perfect state. IT is obscured to the extent that I live the greater part of my life ignorant of IT, of who I really am. This ignorance, constituting the "fall," was previously described.

One of the situations, then, that prevails in the mayic state is this: it appears that there are two entities, my "self" and my "mind." Having convinced me that these are separate and real my ordinary mind proceeds to play endless games with the two concepts. A number of these were described in chapter 1 and we should here restate the situation. My "self" appears to be the representative of my existence. The components of this self—a body, emotions, a mind—must be protected from innumerable, constant threats to which it is subject. Simultaneously, it must gratify its desires and fulfill its needs, whatever these are thought to be. This necessitates possessing, manipulating, and otherwise functioning among objects and conditions of what is interpreted to me as the "world." Early in life I am taught to believe that that component which presides over such matters is my mind (brain). Therefore, my fulfillment in life appears to be dependent, to a very great extent, on my mind. The more fulfillment and gratification I require (and, as we have learned, desires and needs never cease) the more I rely on my mind. Soon, the dependence of my self on my mind is almost total and the subsequent attitude of worship of the mind by the self is that which has been described above. In all of this I fail to perceive that *it is ordinary mind interacting with itself that produces the entire show!*

It is true that ordinary mind does contain a remarkable computer and other elements that enable me to undertake a vast range of activities and function with varying degrees of "competence" in the physical world. The point is that ordinary mind's abilities are confined within the limited dimension that it conceives. But it would have me believe that not for a minute is this the case, that in its noble "search for meaning" it has the capacity to explore and comprehend the most sublime mysteries of the cosmos. It supports this contention with countless theories and "sciences" pertaining to fourth and fifth dimensions, parapsychology, psychic phenomena, extraterrestrial life, and it discusses heaven and hell, God, and infinity with authority. But the reality is that ordinary mind can function only in terms of quantities and qualities. It perceives, discriminates, interprets, and advises according to input that it evaluates as "logical." Illogical input is rejected. Even its abstractions must be derived from what it evaluates as

17

logical input. With logical input ordinary mind performs its functions and advises me of the readout. I interpret this readout as "knowing" and "understanding." I say "I *know*," or "I don't *understand*" such-and-such. But ordinary mind can know (or not know) only in terms of the above-mentioned quantities and qualities; consequently, it can only know *about* things. It can never KNOW; it can never apprehend anything *directly, totally, absolutely*. Direct apprehension, total KNOWING requires the dissolution of the subject-object relationship. There can be no duality of one who knows and a thing that is known; in KNOWING, the knower and the known are *one*.

So while the ordinary mind may discourse endlessly and with great authority and brilliance in all matters, sacred and profane, this all remains perpetual speculation. Operating in the only manner it can—in a subject-object relationship—ordinary mind can purport to distinguish between fantasy and reality, it can discuss God, spirit, and soul, but it can KNOW nothing of such things. When the second man—the "deaf" man—was advised by the Master to "find your self (SELF)," he interpreted this input as "illogical." His ordinary mind dismissed it as being without relevance, without meaning. He heard but he did not UNDERSTAND. The first man, hearing the same words, did not submit them to his ordinary mind for evaluation. He apprehended their meaning *directly*. He comprehended, he KNEW what these words meant because he became *one* with their meaning. He was no longer a self (subject) attempting to apprehend meaning (object). He understood that the situation was not one of an ordinary mind (the Master's) attempting to convey an image to another ordinary mind (his own) but of SELF communicating with itself! If the foregoing sentences are submitted to your ordinary mind, if you must examine and find the logic of the words, you will be "deaf" as was the second man. Only if you apprehend their meaning directly, with Universal Mind, can you UNDERSTAND them. Because a major objective of Yoga practice is the attainment of direct apprehension we shall examine the possibilities of this attainment in much greater detail subsequently.

Shall we, then, dispense with the ordinary mind? Of course not. But we will attempt to view it from a transcendental perspective and realize that it is a temporary agent of the SELF. Ordinary mind is indispensable to our functioning in the physical world. It provides us with the many necessary facts and statistics that we must have to navigate physically, mentally, and emotionally among the objects and conditions of the world. But if we allow ordinary mind to appropriate endless power, to take over, to lead us down the garden path and convince us, over and over again, that it has the capacity to provide ultimate fulfillment, we shall never cease to suffer. When I turn to ordinary mind for counsel in attaining fulfillment I make a very grave error. I am seeking security and peace and I continually turn for instruction in attaining these to an entity that creates a dimension of subjects and objects, of illusionary opposites that maintain for me the constant awareness of insecurity and turmoil. The situation is somewhat akin to asking the fox to guard the chickens. The cry of this generation is "Do your own thing," but it is the ordinary mind that presents the images of what this "thing" and what this "self" should be. Ordinary mind has no more knowledge of the SELF than a single cell has knowledge of the entire organism.

One of the most profound deceptions of the ordinary mind is its illusion of "problem solving." A significant part of our worship of mind is based on its ability to solve, or at least cope with, a multitude of problems, large and small, with which we are continually beset. Mind—valiant and capable ally—evaluates our problems and implements the procedures necessary to resolve them. It can deal with many different types of problems simultaneously. Since hardly an hour passes during which I do not experience one or more problems it is obvious to me that this is another indispensable capacity in which my mind serves. But let us look more closely at this problem solving process. From where do the problems come? I envision them as arising from some source that is external and alien. I have the general impression that people, conditions, and events create a situation—wittingly or unwittingly—that results in my having a problem. (The magnitude of this problem is not important here.) The problem is apprehended by my mind and the problem solving procedure is initiated. In the course of my everyday life it is inconceivable to me that my problems do not arise from "outside" myself. It is unthinkable that the entity that is called upon to cope with and hopefully "solve" the problem—my mind—is the very entity that creates the problem! And yet, under scrutiny from our extra-mayic perspective, this is exactly what we discover. We realize that there are no "outside" problems. The world and nature create not a single perplexity. *My ordinary mind creates them.* This is indeed a startling realization because, as previously stated, we cannot imagine any situation in which our minds—our friends, servants, and advisers in whom we place unqualified trust—would not act in our best interests. Why would my mind deceive me? Why would it create problems with which to frustrate and torment me?

The truth is that the computer aspect of my ordinary mind could not care less about my frustrations and sufferings. It may convince me that it has allied itself with my emotions in such a way that it seeks to promote my experience of those which are "positive" and minimize my experience of those which are "negative." But this is not the reality of the situation. The manner in which the ordinary mind functions entails its dealing with quantities, qualities, facts, statistics. How naïve of us to believe that it is a problem "solver" and *not a problem creator!* The situation is similar to our believing that we shall somehow be able to realize happiness without despair and success without failure. It is the ordinary mind that creates our problems and then, as it elects, goes about coping with or "solving" these problems, all the while programming a host of new problems. Our delusion is that the problems originate somewhere "outside" of us and that, through the ingenuity and resourcefulness of the mind, the problems will be resolved. Occasionally we are even led to envision a time when there will be no more problems. But existence in maya is synonymous with endless problems; *the ordinary mind computer has a problem manufacturer built in.* Just as there is no end to desires, so there is no end to problems. They are eternal.

Two other intriguing aspects of the mayic structure are the illusions of *name* and *time*.

The written and spoken word has great power: the "reality" of the world of objects, conditions, and ordinary mind concepts (all changing, all illusionary) is reinforced each time such things are *named*. We come to believe that when we are able to name an object, person, or condition we somehow KNOW and EXPERIENCE it. But it is this very naming which is largely responsible for creating and reinforcing the subject-object relationship. As long as it appears to me that "I (subject) am looking at the flower" (object) I am prevented from truly KNOWING and EXPERIENCING the flower. We shall have a direct understanding of this later.

Also a basic component in the mayic structure, the element of *time* is programmed into virtually all functions of the ordinary mind computer. Consequently, we find it almost impossible to think in terms that do not include the time dimension. Time (past, present, future) imparts a formidable reality to all objects and conditions of maya. We apprehend *changes* in objects and conditions, and changes appear to transpire in a continuum, a sequence that we designate as "time." Time is an especially potent reinforcer of the value of *action*, for we are taught to accept the proposition "In time, everything comes to he who perseveres" (whatever the forms that his "perseverance" is supposed to take). As with certain other aspects of maya that are manufactured by ordinary mind, time is an important convenience for mayic arrangements. But it is a convenience that turns into a destructive monster when it exerts such influence upon us that we become its slaves.

Birth and death, growth and decay, sunrise and sunset, and the change of the seasons would appear to lend undisputable reality to time. But SELF is ETERNAL. "Eternal" is not something that is born and lives a very long time; "eternal" means *no* birth, *no* death, *no* beginning, *no* end. It simply IS. What is ETERNAL is *timeless*. While the illusion of time reinforces the promise of the conspiracy that "what we do not now have, we shall *someday* have" (the diversionary opiate of "hope"), the truth of the matter is that because SELF is ETERNAL it exists only NOW and can never exist in any place and at any "time" other than NOW. NOW is not to be equated with the "present," as a component of the past-present-future sequence. NOW is NOW. NOW is ALL. NOW is without the qualities of time. There has never been a "past" in which SELF was in any way incomplete and there will never be a "future" in which it will *become* complete! But this truth is contrary to all perceptions of ordinary mind and to all tenets of the mayic conspiracy. It is "illogical" in the extreme and my fellow conspirators want no part of it. They would have me believe that timelessness is a curious, novel conception that may be of interest to theologians, philosophers, and "far-out" physicists, but has no practical relevance to everyday living, to you and me. On the contrary, it has the greatest possible relevance because as long as I do not comprehend that I can exist only NOW I believe the promise that my fulfillment lies in an illusionary "future," providing that I undertake the proper courses of action. Of such courses of action, we have noted, there are no end. The "future" never comes; the "past" never was. These are manufactured conveniences to facilitate the manipulation of mayic conditions. If we make an effort to become very quiet in our bodies and to stop our thoughts for a few moments we may have an inkling that AWARENESS is occurring NOW. Have we ever been AWARE at any time, in any dimension other than NOW? The ordinary mind computer can spew forth all of the "facts" that comprise a "past" but you can be AWARE of these facts only NOW. The ordinary mind computer can summon data from which it projects a "future" but are we AWARE of this future in the "future" or NOW? We do not exist in time. We exist only as SELF. To exist as SELF, NOW, implies utilizing the time component as is necessary on the mayic plane, but not as a *reality* that ensnares us in endless actions to achieve fulfillment in an imaginary "future." We are NOW, complete, perfect, and at peace. SELF-realization is the experiencing of these truths—not in an illusionary past or future but NOW. If we do not have this realization NOW we can never have it.

Let us return to our examination of the "self."

I use the word "self" not only to designate a composite of subjective and objective aspects of my existence—body, senses, emotions, actions, mind—but in reference to an entity that I conceive has some type of form and substance, that is in some way *real*. I may acknowledge its elusiveness but I never question its existence. I identify my "self" with my existence. They appear to be one. After all, could I exist without myself? Yes, I can and I do. And it is imperative that I have some insight into this truth for such an insight will assist me in unlocking one of the stoutest doors of the mayic prison. Although I have accepted my self as synonymous with my existence and have had little reason to question its reality I decide, one day, to examine this self; I will look at it carefully and attempt to determine all I can about its nature. But regardless of the point at which I begin my investigation, regardless of how many different paths I pursue and how "far out" or "far in" I travel, regardless of how simple, complex, subtle, or gross are my investigative techniques, I eventually arrive at only one conclusion: there is no "self," no "me" to examine. An "I" is nowhere to be grasped! I come to realize that my investigation is only ordinary mind investigating itself. I have no self without my mind. I have no separate self, no "I" apart from the one that is manufactured and sustained by ordinary mind. What a fantastic game ordinary mind plays: it creates the impression of a "self" and then proceeds to go in search of it so that it can be examined!

I know myself only as ordinary mind permits me to know myself. I know that I am "I" only when I *think* about "I"—and then only to the extent that ordinary mind provides the pertinent thoughts that it labels "me." Each time I must identify or reidentify myself I am actually manufactured anew. I call upon my mind to furnish the identifying series of statistics. My brain, the ultimate computer, is able, in the smallest fraction of a second, to provide a multitude of such statistics—thought forms that succeed one another with incalculable rapidity—that have been recorded and stored in its banks. Instantaneously, I am presented with my name, address, age, physical characteristics, affiliations, relationships, likes, dislikes, ambitions, and whatever else is required in a particular situation to reestablish or reinforce the "I." (Accompanying emotions are likewise evoked as necessary.) Therefore, "I" exist in relation to the statistics or thoughts that I have about my "self" and *only in relation to these thoughts*.

But the machinations of ordinary mind are even more extensive. It does not limit its construction to a single "I"; any number of "I's" are manufactured! At one end of the "I" spectrum there is my supergood "I," possessing all the qualities that are regarded as virtuous and desirable; at the other end there is the abysmally bad "I" to which are attributed the opposite, objectionable qualities. In between there are all degrees of good and bad "I's." The identities (statistics) of each can be summoned forth in a split second. I like to identify with the good I's that will, through a variety of high-principled undertakings, eventually transform the bad I's into good I's. Since I am continually informed by my fellow conspirators that the transformation of bad into good is highly commendable (it is sometimes known as "self-improvement") I can easily make this a lifelong activity. It is an utterly futile one. "Good," no matter how it is conceived, is eternally the other end of "bad." I recognize "good" only as it is relative to "bad." Therefore, in order to manifest a virtuous, moral, constructive, good self, my unvirtuous, immoral, destructive, bad self must remain alive and well. But being largely ignorant of this, I continue to function as though "self-improvement" is a desirable and attainable objective.

The manner in which ordinary mind undertakes this self-improvement process is fascinating. For example, when I say, "I must lose twenty-five pounds," I am envisioning a bad "I"—a treacherous scoundrel—who, weak and undisciplined, has through its uncontrolled appetites added twenty-five excessive pounds to my physical I. My good I, with whom "I" am now identifying, understands that these extra twenty-five pounds are undesirable. My physical I has conveyed this fact to my good I through the negative, overloaded way it feels. Additionally, my good I has reached this conclusion through its intellect, through facts about the dangers of excessive weight that have come to its attention. At this point my good I loathes both my bad I and my physical I, holding them responsible for the dreadful overweight condition. It knows that it must now confront my bad I, convince it that it must alter its degenerate ways, stop it from seducing my physical I into additional pounds, and, in general, assist my good I in a weight-loss program. What we have here, then, is three I's: there is the physical I (he's the dumb one; all he does is the eating), my bad I (he's the seducer of unsuspecting physical I's; he encourages them to eat themselves into oblivion), and my good I (the noble, clear-thinking I who must rescue my physical I from the clutches of my bad I). My good I considers various approaches to my bad I ranging from logic and reason to harsh discipline. Accordingly, certain measures are implemented (what they are is unimportant). But when lunchtime arrives I eat six doughnuts and a hot fudge sundae! What happened? Well, I decided that I will begin my diet *tomorrow* morning and that I am entitled to "just one more good time." Which "I" is it that has made this decision? What dialogue developed among the three I's? Did my bad I whine, plead, threaten, exhort? Did my good I conclude that a compromise was the best course? Were the doughnuts and sundae needs of my physical I simply overpowering? Did I somehow switch my sympathies and identify with my bad I, casting my good I to the winds? Again, the answers are unimportant here but what is extremely revealing is how these "I" dynamics manifest—how they are involved in much of our thinking and action.

"I's" are manufactured by ordinary mind, invested with identities that make them appear real and set to playing endless games with one another. Our everyday phrases attest to our unquestioning acceptance of this self plurality. One hears expressions such as "I have decided to improve myself." Here we have an "I" who has decided that there is another "I" (myself) that needs to be "improved." The first I is going to work on the second I, as a sculptor molds a piece of clay, until the second I is "improved." And who will make the determination that the project is proceeding satisfactorily—that the first I is correctly improving the second I? Why, an impartial observer: a *third* I, of course! (Unfortunately, we find this observer, this third I, frequently slipping from its position of objectivity and taking an active voice in informing the first I of its inadequacies in improving the second I.) A current popular expression enjoins us to "get it all together." In this case there is a principal self who perceives that an unknown number of additional selves, its charges, have gone astray, become "strung out." This principal "I" is, therefore, proposing that the dispersed selves be brought back into the fold, united with one another and with itself, the principal self. Whatever course is followed to achieve this absurd objective the task will prove extremely trying: for each rebellious self that is returned to wherever the principal self envisions it is supposed to be, the holes in the fence permit several additional dissident selves to escape. The person who is involved in "getting it all together" *never* gets it all together. The best he can hope for is brief moments of respite between escapes. Or we hear, "I think I am going out of my mind." How many selves do we count in this bizarre declaration? Now there is (1) an I who "thinks" about (2) an I who is "going" (3) out of a "mind" that must be in the possession of yet another I ("my"). And who is it that is able to observe and analyze all this that is transpiring among the three I's? Why, a *fourth* I. And it follows that only a *fifth* I could be taking note of the existence of these other four I's; and so on into infinity. Amid all of these I's is there one that is more genuinely my true I? If so, will the real I, the real self please stand up? The REAL SELF will stand up splendidly; indeed, It has never sat down. But It cannot be found in the mayic condition. The numerous I's, mes, and yous are thoughts and concepts of the ordinary mind. Try as we may, we shall find not a trace of a "self" to "get a grip on," or to "improve"!

"Now wait just a moment," protests the reader. "I *see* myself, I *feel* myself, I am *conscious* of myself. Are you really telling me that I do not exist?" Exactly so. The "I" that you are referring to does not exist in the real, ultimate, absolute sense that is totally pertinent to our everyday lives. And what a supremely joyous revelation this is, since it grants instantaneous relief from the bur-

den of caring with all of one's energies for an illusionary "I." You *do see* a physical body, but not a "self."
You *are conscious,* you *are aware* but not of a "self."
The self, the source of delusion and suffering, appears
only when ordinary mind manufactures it. *The existence
of the self is the concept of the self.* The innumerable
"I's" have no reality; they arise and disappear only as
thoughts—thoughts succeeding one another with such
incalculable rapidity that the illusion of a *simultaneity*
manifests. But there can be only one thought, only one
aspect of one self manufactured at any given moment.
When the thought is gone, the I is gone. This can be
confirmed by consciously *interrupting* the flow of
thoughts, by literally "turning them off."

Ordinarily, as we indicated earlier, my thoughts are
incessant and irrepressible. On a perpetual basis they
succeed one another with great force and rapidity. Although I have no knowledge of how and from where
they arise, and where they go when I am no longer
aware of them (the terms "waves," "impulses," "subconscious," etc., are objective designations of men of
science and in no way explain the nature of thoughts
as I actually experience them), they appear to be *my*
thoughts, occurring in *my* mind and requiring *my* attention. I do not suspect this incessant procession of
thoughts; I regard it as natural, as the process of
"thinking." It does not register with me that ordinary
mind, in order to maintain its complete dominance,
deems it essential that my attention be fully and permanently occupied with "thoughts." So the brain, the
thinking machine, the computer that is meant to serve
by furnishing information relevant to specific situations, grossly exceeds its intended function and "takes
over." Unremittingly the thoughts come and go, their
endless modifications come and go, come and go
again, and again, and regardless of their nature, no
matter how preposterous and enslaving they may be I
am committed to devote my energies to each. (We
must again note here that I have no perception whatsoever of a "mind." I am aware only of a thought, an
impression; I *assume* that this thought and those that
precede and follow it are passing through a "mind,"
somewhat as a train travels through a tunnel.)

27

This "thought" process is so firmly established, so automatic, that the direction "Turn off your thoughts" is evaluated by ordinary mind as "illogical" input. "Why," it asks incredulously, "should I want to stop the thoughts when it is the process of thinking that makes everything possible?" Ordinary mind fiercely resists this "illogical" suspension of thoughts (which it is really interpreting as an extraordinary threat) and makes it extremely difficult to execute. Consequently, a concerted effort is required to interrupt the thinking process for even the briefest interval. But if I succeed there is no more "I." There is consciousness but it is not "self" consciousness. There is awareness, but it is not awareness being perceived by an "I." It is awareness only. Awareness alone. AWARENESS. This is not to be confused with "nothingness"; it is a profound state, transcending maya, that manifests when it is unobscured by ordinary mind, by thinking. It is the approach to our REAL state. We shall have much to say of it subsequently. But at this point it would be meaningful for the reader to attempt the application of the "thought suspension" practice. Sitting down in a comfortable position and remaining quiet and relaxed for several minutes without external distractions he should determine what occurs if he is successful in "turning off" his thoughts. There are no special techniques required, no secret knowledge to be applied, and *no specific results to be sought*. It is simply a matter of attempting to experience a brief interval of AWARENESS, of consciousness without thought. Such an experience, however abbreviated, would be highly significant at this point. . . .

But the interval of AWARENESS is now abruptly terminated. Ordinary mind, furious at being transcended for even a moment, bursts upon one's quietude with a raging torrent of thoughts that cannot be restrained. The "I" is recreated; the mayic condition is reestablished. Ordinary mind has made careful note of this threatening transgression. It will be certain to utilize every resource to prevent this practice from being undertaken again. The devices that it employs toward this end are well known to every beginning student of *meditation*.

The reader will have noted certain obvious ambiguities that are involved in this chapter. The fundamental ambiguities—those that pervade the entire discussion —may be expressed as follows: by the very propositions that have been set forth here, is it not ordinary mind that is writing about ordinary mind, and is it not ordinary mind that is reading about ordinary mind? That is, when I, the author, write about ordinary mind is it not *my* ordinary mind that is formulating the thoughts with which to convey this information? And when you, the reader, in following these thoughts gain an insight into the nature of ordinary mind, is this not accomplished through the properties of *your* ordinary mind? Is ordinary mind not a closed circle, an entity that can give the impression of getting "one up" on itself but always remains ordinary mind even in its "one-upsmanship"? And if I realize the value of transcending ordinary mind, of seeking my real SELF, is it not ordinary mind that has arrived at this conclusion? If the nature of ordinary mind is as described in this chapter, why and how would it reach the conclusion to transcend itself?

In responding to these questions let us again cite the example of the Master and his two listeners. By virtue of being a Master, an "enlightened" man, his words issue forth from the SELF. These words are directed to the SELF contained within the two listeners. The ordinary mind of the second man, the "deaf" man, is a closed circle, so completely closed and obscuring SELF to such an extent that the LIGHT of the Master's words is unable to penetrate. The LIGHT rebounds, diffuses, the words are meaningless. But the ordinary mind of the first man has a gap in its enclosure, a chink in its armor. The nature of this aperture and why it should exist in the first man and not in the second will concern us in the next chapter. But the fact that it *is* there permits the LIGHT of the words, their extramayic meaning, to penetrate, to pass through and awaken the sympathetic vibrations of the SELF at which they were directed. Thus, the Master utilizes words as a *tool* of the ordinary mind to convey SELF to SELF. Words constitute a grossly inadequate medium through which to communicate the nature of SELF. Their inadequacy is responsible for the ambiguities with which this discussion is permeated. Words are the product of ordinary mind—the very entity we are attempting to place in a wholly different perspective—and impose the limitations and distortions of their creator. In the above sentence we stated, ". . . to convey SELF to SELF." In reality, there are not two SELVES, an object SELF and a subject SELF. There is only SELF. But the "SELF to SELF" phrase was used because it is more intelligible and at this stage of the study we are involved in an intricate, delicate process: since we must obviously engage the attention of the ordinary mind we will cater to it by programming at least partial "logical input" while simultaneously seeking to transcend it. It is in this context that we are employing concepts and techniques that appear to originate in ordinary mind and to be directed to ordinary mind. Actually, they are being used transcendentally; they originate in and are directed to SELF. The entire preceding discourse on "self," "desire," "action," etc., is designed to confound ordinary mind by appealing to it through its own agents—investigation, analysis, and dialectics. In consciously turning ordinary mind upon itself, through serious examination of our "self" delusion, we cause cracks to appear in the mayic structure. The more we continue to question the nature of ordinary mind, even though it appears to be ordinary mind that is doing the questioning, the greater the possibility of placing it ultimately in the position that it is meant to occupy, and the more hopeful the prospect of being extricated from those entanglements of it that would hold us a perpetual prisoner. When there are sufficient breaches in its structure the entire house of cards that it has manufactured topples. UNIVERSAL MIND, SELF remains.

"But I don't know if I want that to happen," declares the reader. "What will become of me if the structure *should* disintegrate?" In response to this we must ask, "*Who* is expressing the anxiety?" The SELF has no fear. It is ordinary mind that is concerned about the "I" it maintains; it is ordinary mind creating the fiction that something will be "lost," that one's worst fears of danger and threat will be realized should it cease to occupy its place of unquestioned dominance.

Another "self-preservation" question takes the form of a peculiar concern for one's prison: "What would become of society if *everybody* wanted to transcend his ordinary mind?" Imagine a man who awakens to find his apartment house on fire and those who reside in it suffocating from smoke inhalation and racked with pain from the heat. The firemen respond and provide a rescue net. Rather than jump into the net, this man, with flames licking at him from all sides, elects to engage in a debate with his would-be rescuers as to the fate of the burning house if all within should escape!

Returning to the problem of ambiguity: our attempt to transcend ordinary mind has not been confined to analysis. We have taken direct action (or, more properly, nonaction) toward this end. When we sat quietly for a brief interval and "turned off" our thoughts we experienced no sense of "loss" or "fear." If anything, the sensation was one of having *found* or *rediscovered* a dimension of our existence of which we are usually ignorant. We have barely touched on this state of SELF and there are no other conclusions that we shall draw at this point. We refer to that technique of "turning off the thoughts" again here because it enables us, if we so choose, to simply dismiss whatever ambiguities may prove inhibiting and conduct a *direct* approach to the transcending of ordinary mind.

The response, then, to the ambiguity encountered in this presentation is twofold: (1) ambiguity (contradiction, duplexity) will work to our advantage as described above; (2) it can be disregarded when it proves excessively troublesome and various practices can be undertaken that provide *direct* experience of the indicated objectives.

Now, the material of these first two chapters is concerned, primarily, with the presentation of a perspective of life as it is experienced in maya. Additionally, there have been inferences that it is possible to achieve liberation from the mayic bonds. But before pursuing the implications of "liberation" it will be well for us to review the situation, to summarize those conditions that we experience from moment to moment on the mayic plane: we exist in a dimension of constant threat and danger. We are beset on all sides by endless problems that, in our delusion, we attempt to resolve with the very entity that creates them. We seek to KNOW and UNDERSTAND but cannot because we are eternally separated, in a subject-object relationship, from that which we would KNOW. Through a universal conspiracy we accept these situations as "the natural course of events," as "life." Hypnotized by the self-appropriated authority of ordinary mind, immersed and believing in not only one but many "selves" that ordinary mind manufactures and maintains, we subscribe unquestioningly to its illusive propositions. Among these fantasies the doctrine of desire-action-fulfillment convinces us that it is natural and necessary to strive for happiness, success, pleasure, and security, that such elusive objectives can be achieved through the right kind of action and that somehow our achievements can be made permanent. Thus, dutifully complying with the party line of the conspiracy, we spend our lives experiencing incessant desires that compel us to undertake the incessant actions dictated for their fulfillment. But because our desires are interminable, because our actions can never truly satisfy these desires, and because we seek what is ultimate and permanent in a state where only constant impermanence and fluctuation obtains, we suffer. We suffer not only throughout this lifetime but throughout an infinite number of lifetimes.

How shall we escape from this prison of maya?

When shall we awaken from those illusions that promote perpetual anxiety and experience the only reality wherein peace and fulfillment lie—the SELF?

Chapter 3

Dis-illusionment:
Exposing the Conspiracy

More than anything, it is, paradoxically, sheer weariness that causes the ignorant, deaf, sleeping being to "awaken." At some point, after innumerable lifetimes of suffering, of countless actions undertaken in a fruitless quest for fulfillment, the sleeping being experiences an event that acts as the final straw. Whatever this event may be (and it may be anything), it acts as the precipitating cause of his questioning the promises of fulfillment that have been eternally held out to him by the conspirators. He begins to mistrust the ways that he has been told he must follow for the attainment of security and peace. Thus a pinhole of light appears in the curtain; the sleeping man begins to stir. Continued questioning results in greater unrest that intensifies and accelerates the awakening process.

The initial stages of awakening frequently generate a profound conflict. The awakened being functions in a condition in which he is still largely subject to the dominance of ordinary mind and governed by the principles of the conspiracy but in which there is a partial cognition of SELF. The resultant turbulence of being subject to two forces, of existing simultaneously in what is experienced as two very different dimensions, usually makes for a difficult period. Having once awakened, a man may intermittently nap but he cannot return to his undisturbed sleep. Deep stirrings, welcome or unwelcome, will continue to prod this man so that he is literally pushed and pulled into an ever-widening recognition of the conspiracy, of the illusion. An expression of this conflict can be found throughout the scriptures of both East and West. Jacob, Moses, David, Paul, and St. John of the Cross are familiar examples of those who articulated their distress in this situation.

The awakened man eventually understands that he is in the position of a traveler plodding along a path that is perceived only as through a glass darkly. He trudges forth, frequently stumbling, continually encountering obstacles and confused by incessant adversities. He may briefly rest, he may even reverse his direction temporarily, but ultimately he is committed to resume his forward movement. Although he has a sense of destination and may, if the light is just right, catch an occasional view of the road ahead, his vision is largely obscured. Sooner or later it becomes evident that the services of a guide are required.

The *Guru* is the guide on the path.

Many paths lead to the SELF. All have their respective Gurus. Each age, each culture has developed systems of SELF-realization. The most cursory perusal of philosophy and metaphysics discloses numerous such systems. Why an individual should be attracted to a particular system and elect to traverse one path in preference to another is a matter of inclination, of tendency, of natural disposition, of physical circumstances, and of the teacher, the Guru who may be involved.

The major schools of Indian philosophy are unique in that they are not opposed or even contradictory to one another. They simply approach the cognition of SELF from different vantage points. Of these schools the two that are acknowledged to treat SELF-realization in the most comprehensive manner are *Vedanta* (the end of wisdom), which concerns itself with the nature and state of SELF, and *Yoga*, which presents those techniques that enable the seeker to attain *direct experience* of the SELF. This book is concerned primarily with Yoga.

The many paths that have developed as variations of the major systems of SELF-realization (and it is interesting to note that SELF-realization means, literally, "making the SELF *real*") all have their Gurus. The word "Guru" has become very popular in the Western world and while little less than a decade ago a Guru evoked a most alien image—some strange, scantily clothed *fakir,* ready to hypnotize the unsuspecting Westerner, subject him to degenerate pagan rituals and rob him of his reason and possessions—it is suddenly very "in," very fashionable to speak about "Gurus." Consequently, the term is being applied not only to a large number of people who have anything to say about philosophy and metaphysics, but has been extended to include a multitude of teachers in all subjects: artists, writers, musicians, and even entertainers, professional sportsmen, and drug pushers. It is startling and tragic to hear an interview with a drug addict in which he describes how he was initially "turned on" by his "LSD Guru"! This may be the ultimate example of a misnomer in the history of language.

While the term "Guru" has been used in the East— particularly India—to denote respect for one's spiritual teacher (regardless of the teacher's attainments), in the most venerable of the Yoga *shastras* (scriptures) a "Guru" denotes either a totally enlightened or a highly evolved spiritual being who, in one form or another, imparts instruction and guidance. In this book "Guru" is used only in the latter context. We do not apply the term to avant-garde poets, to the Yoga teacher at the local YWCA who may be two chapters ahead of her students in the textbook, or to most of the visiting Indians who appear intent on competing with one another to determine who can establish the most branch offices or the most *ashrams* the quickest. While many of these Hindus may have something to say that deserves attention and consideration, they are not Gurus (dispellers of ignorance) in the classical sense.

The true Guru is a dis-illusioner. Throughout the ages he has blown the whistle on the conspiracy; he has explained the nature of maya. Different periods, cultures, and attitudes require different types of whistles and different methods of blowing them. But essentially Gurus address themselves to those in the society—whatever their stations—who have developed "ears to hear," who have "awakened," who seek guidance on the path. The teachings and techniques of the Gurus take many forms ranging from the doctrine of love and humility as espoused by Jesus to the slap in the face by the Zen Roshi, to being shown how to get out of your own way and let things function naturally (the path of the Taoist), to the application of breath control and *asanas* that comprise the system of *Hatha Yoga*.

The following is the essence of what is transmitted by the Guru of the path with which this book is concerned:

1. The SELF, God, Brahma, is ALL; there is none other. SELF is pure, spotless, unconditional, infinite, eternal, and transcends "existence" and "non-existence"; hence IT is REAL. Fulfillment lies in the uncovering and recognition of SELF.

2. A man/woman suffers without end as long as he/she lives in ignorance of SELF. This ignorance is equated with the state of *maya*, illusion. All in maya is transient, impermanent, and, in this sense, *unreal*.

3. In his ignorance man identifies with body, senses, and mind and attaches himself to the things and conditions of the world, attempting to possess, manipulate, and function among them in ways that will result in his happiness and fulfillment. As a consequence he is confined to an existence of subject-object relationships that appear to transpire in a dimension of "time."

4. In his ignorance man falls under the spell of his servant, the usurper, ordinary mind. Ordinary mind manufactures multitudinal "I's" whose appetites require endless gratification. Consequently, interminable "action" is undertaken to satisfy the desires of the manufactured "I's."

5. Because SELF is in all things and all things are of SELF (a fact that is obscured by the incessant activity of the faculties of ordinary mind), all things become a path to SELF.

In the above context the function of the Guru becomes twofold: (1) he exposes the conspiracy that prevails on the mayic plane by revealing the nature of ordinary mind; (2) according to the Yoga that is involved he provides the techniques and guidance that lead to the SELF. These are ongoing processes that continue on different levels as long as the Guru-disciple relationship is in effect. But it is a relationship that requires the most delicate judgment on the part of the Guru, for, in its course, the student comes to regard his Guru with great reverence and it is not unusual that this reverence develops into a type of fanatical worship. All the while, the Guru is aware of a most vital and profound truth: *he, the Guru, cannot impart enlightenment or liberation; he can only point the way. The real giver of wisdom, the One who truly enlightens is the GURU WITHIN.* The art of the Guru lies in pushing the disciple from without so that the GURU may pull from within. The fact that the true GURU is *within* is a most difficult one to convey to the disciple, especially in his initial stages of awakening. He is inclined to view the external, physical Guru as the repository of all of the virtues and miraculous powers that his romantic fantasy can impute. But the Guru knows better. He may accept the position of awe in which he is held but only if he can employ it as a device to convey that what the disciple is doing in using him, the Guru, as the object of worship is externalizing SELF and projecting the GURU WITHIN onto the physical form of the Guru. So, as often as the disciple would seek wisdom, fulfillment, and peace with his ordinary mind, that is, in the world of objects, people, and conditions, the Guru will turn him back upon himself, direct him to seek his objectives "within." Rather than attempting to establish a protracted Guru-disciple relationship, it is the Guru's function to have the disciple realize in the shortest possible time that the GURU is within and that he, the physical Guru, is extraneous, that, indeed, he can actually represent an *obstacle* to the disciple's liberation.

It must be reiterated that in all of this we are using the term "Guru" in its classical context, denoting either a fully SELF-realized being or one who is highly evolved. The fact is, however, that relative to the world population there is a very small number of such fully realized beings. Of these, only a fraction act in the capacity of a Guru who undertakes the *direct* instruction of students, and of these, the number of true Gurus of Yoga who have journeyed to the Western world are very, very few. Therefore, the situation currently prevailing is that an awakening man who is attracted to one of the paths of Yoga *may* find a *teacher* who is able to convey to him, in an adequate manner, the principles of that path. But the possibility of this man finding a Yoga Guru in the classical meaning of the word is exceedingly small; this holds true not only in the countries of the Western world but in India as well. The difficulty is compounded when one understands that even having encountered a being who is ostensibly a true Guru the seeker cannot know whether this being will be *his* Guru. A relationship of the most subtle nature—usually extending over a significant period of time—must be established between the teacher and the student before each can determine if the teacher is the true Guru for this particular disciple.

We noted above that only a fraction of the SELF-realized beings undertake to act in the capacity of Gurus. To the uninformed reader this information is often puzzling. "Why," he wonders, "are not *all* enlightened beings making this world a better place in which to live by sharing their knowledge openly and widely with all mankind and by personally instructing the greatest possible number of interested students?" This person does not understand the purpose and function of the Guru nor does he comprehend those methods through which wisdom is conveyed. Even the awakening man, still largely dominated by the ordinary mind and still believing that fulfillment is somehow connected to the plane of objects and conditions, is frequently inclined to envision the Guru as a type of social or political figure—one who is concerned with resolving "worldly" problems and bettering living conditions. Such "worldly" improvements *may* result from the teachings of certain Gurus but they must be understood as by-products of these teachings. Gurus are not concerned with increasing the disciple's odds for getting what he thinks he wants out of life. True Gurus are *uncompromising liberators;* the ordinary mind can seldom countenance or comprehend their transcendental teachings. The student who undertakes the practice of Yoga in the hope that this practice will improve his lot in life is not yet ready for Yoga.

The Western world is currently in the throes of Gurumania. The demand for Gurus is producing, among other phenomena, bizarre, self-styled, self-proclaimed "Gurus," as well as numerous visitors from India whose motives and "Guru" abilities should be closely examined by potential "disciples." The author has personal knowledge of hundreds of seekers who are dissipating their precious life-force by running from one teacher to another, from one retreat or *ashram* to another, from one state or country to another, hoping to encounter a Guru. Some of these seekers are involved in a genuine quest for instruction; many are looking for a being whom they have romantically preconceived as a sort of superman, someone who will "turn them on," "bend their minds," send them on a "far-out trip" or impart enlightenment with a magic gesture, *mantram,* or ritual. All are subject to the Guru myth. But the fact that there *is* this driving desire to discover an external Guru contains an essential implication: the seeker presupposes that there is knowledge and wisdom to be acquired that he does not possess. Such is not the case. The seeker does, now and always, possess what he believes he is in quest of, and as we have stated, the Guru's function is to turn the disciple into himself so that he, the disciple, comes to know with the deepest possible conviction that his guidance on the path unfolds from *within.*

If, instead of expending the vast amounts of effort and time in what is generally an unproductive search for the external Guru, the awakening man and all those who seek guidance would understand that such guidance must be sought within themselves, they would soon find that they are indeed being instructed by the only Guru—the internal GURU. We have suggested that the possibility of encountering a true Guru is exceedingly remote and, moreover, that such an encounter must not be considered as essential. The position that *should* be taken by those in the Western world who are attracted to Yoga and are, in some degree, engaged in Yogic practices, is that at some point in their studies a Guru, embodied in a physical form, *may* appear but that it is actually of no consequence whether he does or does not; the most sublime wisdom that he imparts will be pale in comparison with that which is continually available from the ultimate GURU within.

How does the student evoke this internal instruction? We have noted that it is the function of the external Guru to "push" so that the GURU may "pull." The physical Guru utilizes various methods—some of which have been outlined above—to implement the "push"; he acts as a type of catalyst. The propositions and techniques of this book (and other similar sources of instruction to which the student may be attracted) attempt to provide this same catalytic action. Each time the Yoga techniques presented herein are seriously applied by the student they "push" him within, they open him more and more to the illumination of the GURU.

Once understanding that the GURU guides from within, the student learns how to listen for this guidance. His listening is done with an inner ear that gradually becomes attuned and sensitive to the inner voice. In the initial stages the catalyst, the "push," is implemented and the guidance received primarily during "practice sessions." These sessions may consist of the application of prescribed techniques such as *asanas, pranayama, mantra, yantra* (any and all of which comprise the "push"), and the guidance is received during regulated periods of meditation. At times the instruction is readily available; at times it is slow in coming. But the student understands this pattern and waits patiently because he knows it *will* be forthcoming.

The form that the inner instruction takes cannot be articulated; it is subtle, sublime, and transcends altogether that knowledge which is sought by ordinary mind. This is Knowledge and Understanding of an entirely different type—not of the transient but of the ETERNAL. As the inner voice continues to be heard the student becomes increasingly SELF-reliant; he seeks less and less direction from people and conditions of the world—the world that is interpreted to him by ordinary mind and the senses. The mayic conspiracy, ingeniously camouflaged during innumerable lifetimes, now becomes more and more obvious.

Eventually, the disciple is able to contact the GURU almost at will and ultimately he perceives that he is receiving guidance not only during practice sessions but continually, every moment, regardless of where he is or what he is doing. The GURU pulls and guides the disciple to SELF. When the self of the disciple merges with SELF, when Yoga or reintegration is achieved, the GURU is no more.

> *Without leaving his house,*
> *one can know everything*
> *that is necessary.*
> *Without leaving himself,*
> *one can grasp all wisdom.*
> —Lao Tzu

Chapter 4

The Guru's Guru:
Patanjali and the Eight Steps of Yoga

According to Yogic scriptures, the science of Yoga dates from the most remote antiquity. (See, for example, IV, 1 of the *Bhagavad Gita*.) It is revealed anew to each age (an "age" consisting of at least a millennium), and in each new revelation its techniques are adjusted according to the emotional, intellectual, and spiritual capacity of that age so as to make its application practical. Yoga, in many of its forms, is currently being revealed on a large scale to the Western world and it may very well be that just as in the first century of this era Buddhism was introduced into China from India and took root there, so is Yoga now taking significant root in and profoundly influencing the Western world.

The science of Yoga postulates the existence of the state of SELF, wherein perfection, permanence, and peace obtain. It is this state and *only this state that is recognized as real*. Yoga proposes that the solution to the problem of ignorance, of not knowing who we are, of continual suffering through infinite lifetimes, is the reidentification or conscious union of what we now, at this moment, envision as our composite "self" with the ultimate reality of SELF. This union is Yoga. The Sanskrit phrase employed to describe the experience of this union is *sat-chit-ananda:* perfect being, direct knowledge, eternal bliss. Yoga reestablishes us in our original state; it is the reintegration with this state that each individual soul—knowingly or unknowingly—seeks. The comfort, happiness, and fulfillment that each self longs to experience and that motivates all of its actions is but a gross projection of *sat-chit-ananda.*

SELF-realization is not something that is to be acquired, something to be gained through the acquisition of any object or quality that the self deems desirable or necessary. SELF is our original state, our true nature, and, maya to the contrary, we could never be separated from SELF, the source of our existence, for a split second. Consequently, there is nothing to be acquired; rather, Yoga might be described as the process of *divesting*—divesting oneself of those layers or veils that confine him to an existence in which his identification with a body, senses, and mind gives rise to the illusion of a self that is real. The disengagement from illusion, resulting in the reemergence of SELF, is accomplished, in Yoga, in a series of stages each consisting of certain prescribed practices.

"Yoga" is a word now applied to a maze of activities currently in vogue in the Western world and we find a multitude of instructors, both Western and Eastern, teaching widely divergent practices under the general heading of "Yoga." Because many unknowledgeable "teachers" are instructing Yogic practices out of the context of the particular Yoga system to which they belong the student is applying them in an extremely fragmented manner. It has become difficult for the interested layman, or even for the serious student, to gain a comprehensive perspective of Yoga, to discern the common denominator or unifying principle that underlies the many and diverse techniques characterized as "Yogic."

For example, on the campus of a university we encounter several students who are chanting Sanskrit syllables and we are informed that they are practicing

Yoga; a business executive tells us that in the course of his daily business activities he is applying the principles of Yoga; an elderly lady is seated in a cross-legged position gazing at the flame of a candle and we learn that she is practicing Yoga; a well-known concert artist is photographed standing on his head and we read that he practices Yoga. Are all these people really practicing Yoga? If so, what is the relationship of these diverse techniques? Why choose one and not another? Are these valid practices that lead to the designated objectives? There is an authoritative source to which we may turn not only for answers to these questions but for clarification of the entire theory and practice of Yoga.

In approximately the second century B.C. there lived in India a man named Patanjali. Although nothing is known of his life, Patanjali has provided us with the earliest known written, comprehensive synthesis of Yoga. This appears in the form of a series of brief statements known as "sutras" (threads), or sometimes "aphorisms" of Patanjali. This work is monumental; it is so brilliant and incisive that it usually heads all Yoga bibliographies and there is no Yoga Guru who does not consider Patanjali as *his* Guru. We must conclude that if such a precise and enduring synthesis could have been produced several centuries before Christ, the Yoga practices that Patanjali synthesized must indeed be extremely ancient.

While a historical perspective of Yoga can be of interest, and a study of the *shastras*—the *Vedas, Upanishads, Puranas*—can be additive, knowledge of the Patanjali sutras is indispensable to the serious Yoga student. In this chapter we are concerned with the section of the Patanjali sutras that presents the eight "steps" or "stages" of Yoga. This eight-step structure is accepted by all qualified Yoga instructors as the definitive frame of reference for the theory and practice of Yoga. In examining this structure we shall begin with the final step—the eighth—and proceed in a reverse order.

(8) Samadhi

The eighth step, Samadhi, represents the attainment

of Yoga, wherein reintegration and ultimate union are *experienced*. Here, one's original nature is reclaimed and it is "known"—known not intellectually, not by thinking or through discrimination, but known *directly*. This is the state of sat-chit-ananda, the individual self (*jiva*) being absorbed in Universal Mind, SELF.

(6) and (7) Dharana and Dhyana

Samadhi cannot be attained as long as the agitation generated by ordinary mind persists. It is only when this agitation abates that we begin to perceive the state beyond ordinary mind. The scriptural imagery used to describe this situation is a disturbance in a pool filled with pure, clear water. The ripples formed on the surface by any agitation keeps one from seeing to the bottom of the pool; he sees only the ripples. The moment the ripples are stilled, vision to the bottom is clear. The activity produced by thoughts is comparable to the ripples that prevent us from seeing what lies beneath. Patanjali actually defines Yoga as "the cessation of mental distractions." Therefore, the five steps immediately preceding Samadhi are directly concerned with bringing the mind and senses under control.

The sixth and seventh steps, Dharana and Dhyana, are two stages of intensive concentration, of gradually learning to restrict the mind's activities by focusing upon a single point for a comfortable interval. In the sixth step the student selects such a point; this may be an object, an image, a sound—anything upon which the full faculties of the mind may be focused. He performs the prescribed preliminaries (described subsequently) and then begins to fix his mind upon the selected point. The theory is that this fixation will reduce, discourage, and ultimately prevent the arising of distractions. Invariably, however, the initial stages of this practice prove to be fraught with repeated interruptions. The dynamics of this interruption have been mentioned in chapter 2 where we attempted to turn off the mind. The interruption process is so well established that it is designated as an actual "step" by Patanjali. In other words, he cites the fact that the attention will wander in beginning concentration as a necessary stage, i.e., Dharana: interrupted fixation. But, with sustained practice, this stage evolves into steady, *uninterrupted* fixation of the seventh step, Dhyana. Now the subject-object relationship dissolves and the student assumes the form and essence of the object of his concentration. During these two stages of concentration increasingly deeper states of *knowing* are experienced; the veils of illusion are penetrated successively and the student comes to have a progressively more profound understanding of the nature of self and of the various planes of existence. When, through continued practice, unwavering attention is achieved and the thinking process may be suspended at will, ordinary mind can be transcended. Then, the point upon which the mind has been fixed, dissolves. This dissolution constitutes dispersal of the final mist that still obscures Samadhi.

(5) Pratyahara

This step concerns the *senses*. One cannot successfully quiet his thoughts and accomplish the one-pointed concentration objectives of the sixth and seventh steps if the various senses are permitted to function in their usual way. Their activities create constant impressions which, in the attempted practice of concentration, prove highly distracting. Consequently, prior to beginning the concentration practice, Pratyahara, the fifth step, calls for the conscious withdrawal of the senses into a temporary limbo. Withdrawal and deactivation of the senses is itself a form of concentration. In the initial stages patient practice is required to render the senses senseless.

(4) Pranayama

The concentration required in steps five, six, and seven is facilitated by the regulation of breathing. The manner in which one breathes has an immediate and direct influence on his thoughts. Erratic, irregular, obstructed breathing promotes restlessness; slow, quiet, rhythmic breathing retards the flow of thoughts and has a generally quieting effect on the organism. The techniques through which breathing is regulated and ultimately suspended comprise Pranayama, the fourth step.

(3) Asana

A practice session that consists of Pranayama, followed by an extended period of concentration, requires a physical position in which the body can remain quiet, at ease, compact, and in an attitude of complete awareness for the necessary interval. If the body is uncomfortable and forced to move, to adjust itself, during concentration the mind is disturbed; if it does not have a firm base, deep concentration will be difficult. In designating Asana (comfortable, steady posture) as the third step, Patanjali is referring to one of the various folded-leg seated positions that fulfills these requirements. With the body seated motionless and at ease in a cross-legged or Lotus posture—Sukhasana, Siddhasana, Padmasana—the practice of Pranayama and concentration can be undertaken.

(1) and (2) Yamas and Niyamas

These first two steps are moral, ethical, and health guidelines for living. Each step consists of a group of five such guidelines.

The Yamas are injunctions ("Thou shalt *not*"); specifically they prohibit violence, stealing, lying, greed, sensuality. These injunctions can be understood as obvious laws of conduct with which the aspiring Yogi would attempt to comply. But this is a superficial interpretation, for the Yamas are to be applied by the Yogi not only in a moral context but in a much more personal manner. Each Yama must be given careful consideration as it pertains to his development and unfolding, to his perception of SELF. For example, the injunction against *violence* is understood not only in its gross meaning of not murdering or injuring any living thing but of *not wanting* to murder or injure, of the awareness of one's own actions and patterns to the extent that he is eventually able to prevent the arising of the *thought* or *image* of violence. Similarly, the injunction against *lying* implies not only the obvious, but extends to the more subtle concept of *deception*. It requires great life-force to engage in deception, especially when it must be sustained; the one-pointedness objective of Yoga concentration cannot be achieved under such circumstances. And so with each of the

Yamas. *Greed* must be seen in not only the obvious context, but as a seducer that, in requiring ever-increasing acquisition and possession, holds the self captive in the trap of attachment. *Sensuality,* the conscious quest for pleasure, must be carefully moderated. Experience of pleasure is a powerful opiate. As is the case with greed, pleasure begets the need for additional pleasure without end. We have already noted this process in earlier chapters. Here, again, the life-force invested in the quest for pleasure is enormous. The student must learn how, in his endless pursuit of pleasure in the external world, *he is really seeking SELF,* so that he may turn this outward search inward.

The five Niyamas are *qualities to be cultivated:* purity, simplicity, contentment, repeated affirmation (of SELF), sustained resolve (to achieve Yoga). As with the Yamas, the Niyamas must be interpreted in both the obvious and the more profound ways. *Purity* denotes physical and mental cleanliness; it includes attention to diet and to all matters affecting the well-being of the *body* as well as to whatever the student perceives leads to *mental* contamination: his environment, social life, work, etc.

The second of the Niyamas, *simplicity,* suggests simplicity in the student's living habits, but on the deeper level it implies development of the ability to discern those patterns of thinking and action that *complicate* his life, that reinforce his attachments to people, objects, and conditions as sources of true fulfillment. *Contentment* means not only being satisfied with exactly what one is and has *now,* but cultivating the understanding that one always has exactly what he needs and *is* everything that it is necessary for him to be.

Repeated affirmation (of SELF) is comprised of certain practices that so affirm. These are performed silently and continually, without effort, during all of the Yogi's activities. We shall learn of these later. *Sustained resolve* is cultivating the ability to remember that one is practicing Yoga. This may seem to be a peculiar dedication, but we have already mentioned, and all beginning Yoga students will recognize, the rapidity with which the most sincere resolutions pertaining to the inward journey are forgotten. We pointed out that even when a man is deeply impressed with the instruction that he must "find himSELF" he can become oblivious to this information within a matter of minutes. And if, at some point in his life, he *does* decide to undertake the inward journey his pursuit can be of a most spasmodic nature, often suspended for months or even years at a time! "I know I should practice but . . ." (fill in any one or more of several thousand diversions that can be manufactured by ordinary mind for "self" protection). In cultivating *sustained resolve* the student is required to continually attend to his Yoga practice, gradually weakening the diversionary tactics of ordinary mind.

Although five injunctions and five qualities for cultivation are specified in the Yamas and Niyamas it is obvious that the actual number of each that might be listed is many times five. However, if the student attends to the ten that *are* specified he develops the kind of discrimination and perception that extends to all other qualities.

The Yamas and Niyamas are ultimately articles for disengagement and nonattachment. It is most important to understand that what is involved in these first and second steps is not only physical, mental, moral, and ethical conduct but an essential conservation of life-force. This is converted into energy that is employed to great advantage in the various practices of the additional six steps. From the first and second steps we gain the strength, energy, and discrimination that are required. Yoga is not an easy path; it is often described as "the way of the hero," necessitating sustained dedication and strength—physical, emotional, and mental—in order to pursue the study. The Yamas and Niyamas are largely responsible for developing these qualities.

Let us review the eight steps.

Steps one and two provide the practicing Yogi with the guidelines for all aspects of conduct in his life and impart inspiration and life-force to participate in Yoga practice.

In the third step the Yogi assumes that seated posture in which he can remain with ease, motionless, for whatever periods of time are required.

In the fourth step he regulates his breathing.

In the fifth step he retracts his senses and proceeds, through the concentration techniques of the sixth and seventh steps, to penetrate more and more deeply into the nature of all things.

The seven steps culminate in the eighth, Samadhi, ultimate union or Yoga, wherein individual consciousness is reintegrated with the cosmic or Universal Consciousness.

For explanation purposes we have been applying the words "step" and "stage" to the Patanjali structure. But we must note that in the actual practice of Yoga a number of these "steps" are engaged in simultaneously, or nearly simultaneously. For example, steps one and two, pertaining to conduct, are an intrinsic part of the everyday life of the student; whatever the activities in which he finds himself involved he applies the principles of the Yamas and Niyamas. In his practice session he can usually assume the proper seated posture and regulate his breathing within a few minutes. Then, depending upon his previous attainments he may be able to effect the withdrawal of his senses rather quickly, eliminate elementary concentration, and pass directly into deep meditation, Dhyana. Therefore, it is possible that the student may be encompassing several "steps" simultaneously, or moving too quickly among them to accurately deliniate them as "stages." This is why the words "limb" and "fold" are sometimes applied to the Patanjali structure, suggesting a *simultaneity* or *near simultaneity* of practices rather than an absolute step-wise development.

For further clarification we should also note here that the word "Yoga" denotes both the *procedures for achieving the goal and the goal itself*. Knowledge of this fact should dispel the confusion that can arise when the novice hears that someone is "practicing Yoga." What is meant is that the practitioner is applying the *techniques* of Yoga—asana, pranayama, mantra, dhyana, etc.—to achieve union, the ultimate *objective* of Yoga.

PART II

The Ways Within

In whatever way a human being shall
seek Me, in that way can he find Me.
The paths are many, but ultimately,
all come to Me.

—Krishna to Arjuna (*Bhagavad Gita*)

Introduction

I may seek to discover SELF in what I perceive as
"divinely inspired" entities—the Mona Lisa, the Taj
Mahal, the Mass in B Minor—but if I do not know that
SELF is to be found in the dust beneath my feet I am
yet wholly in the dark. Nothing is devoid of SELF.
Through ITS agents, it creates, preserves, and dissolves
all. Therefore, since God, Brahma, Universal Mind, the
Absolute, the Supreme Being is present in all things,
since all persons, objects, and conditions are manifestations of IT, we may conclude that each of these
manifestations constitutes a potential path to SELF.
Each may become an avenue of Yoga.

Those attributes and qualities that exist within "me"
and that I regard as belonging to my "self" are also
such avenues; they are but reflections of the SELF. I
can unite my love with Cosmic Love; I can trace my
intelligence to Cosmic Intelligence; I can perceive my
body as a microcosm of the Universal Body. Each individual has evolved, and continues to develop in a different way. Simply put, people are different and various qualities (*gunas*) are present and active in each
person in different proportions. Therefore, while one

man finds that his intellectual qualities predominate, another leans decidedly toward mysticism, and a third is predisposed toward the devotional life. Still others are preoccupied with the body, are "physical" in nature. As the natural consequence of this fact—that people are different—various types or systems of Yoga have evolved, permitting each individual to utilize his predominating tendencies to achieve reintegration.

Although the systems of Yoga are numerous and subdivisions within these systems have developed, it is unlikely that any person of the Western world who is drawn to Yoga would find it necessary to become familiar with more than six major systems which, through the centuries, have emerged as those which have attracted the greatest number of people. These are: Bhakti, Jnana, Karma, Raja, Laya, Hatha. The different techniques emphasized by each system will be described in the following pages. We shall also indicate how these different systems have evolved as developments or extensions of the original limbs of Patanjali. Subsequent to his study of these pages, the reader should be able to recognize various Yogic practices that he may encounter as techniques basic to a particular system or as the development of a particular limb. An overall perspective of the relationship of one Yoga to another will also be gained.

The type of Yoga and the methods of practice that are instructed to achieve its objectives are dependent on the nature of the teacher. Some teachers are strict traditionalists, others are innovators; so that even while remaining within the Patanjali structure, the presentation of the Yoga systems we shall explore in this book may vary according to the methods of the instructor.

Chapter 1

Bhakti Yoga:
Reunion Through Devotion

Bhakti Yoga is a path for those whose natures are devotional, who are naturally disposed to give of themselves, who experience outpourings of love toward all mankind, who are drawn to be of service to their fellow humans. Such individuals have the emotional capacity to *feel* deeply and can direct these strong emotions into that intense devotional practice which results in identification with and absorption into the Absolute through the quality of love.

The Yogic concept of deep devotion is not essentially different from that with which we are familiar in the various religions of the West. There is a constant awareness of the principle of Love pervading all things. That symbol or image chosen as the representation of the Supreme Being is ever-present in the consciousness of the Bhakta. While profoundly "religious," the Bhakti Yogi's worship is not overt. For the most part his practice is conducted silently within himself and his worship is performed in privacy rather than in a group situation. The overriding theme of Bhakti Yoga is that whatever the object of worship, it must always pervade the mind and heart of the Bhakta.

In the beginning stage of his practice the devotee *anticipates* his eventual identification with the chosen symbol of Love; gradually, through practice and faith, he grows certain that this identification will actualize. The process is one of purification and transformation. The gross love of the Bhakta for things and people is, through constant contemplation, refined and purified so that he comes to perceive and identify with the source, the essence of Love. Implicit in this God-consciousness of the Bhakta is the practice of self-surrender. There can be no perception of SELF when self is present. Therefore, the Bhakta offers whatever he conceives of as his "self" and all activities associated with this self to that which is the object of his worship. This he also performs continuously.

Bhakti is a form of Yoga that the ancient seers pronounced fit for all, and it was described as the simplest of the major Yogas. All were qualified to embark upon this path to liberation. Such a pronouncement was meant as an incentive not only for those who were of a devotional nature but for those who were of the uneducated, poor, and otherwise deprived classes. The power of love was known in the East at a very early date and it was recognized that even abbreviated, wavering attempts to surrender the self, to worship the chosen entity, brought about remarkable transformations in the individual's nature.

Certain of the scriptures provide a general structure for the practice of Bhakti but the rituals and deities indicated in this structure are so firmly fixed in the context of Indian culture that it is not altogether practical for most readers of this book. However, we can adapt the essential practices that are prescribed, through substitution. The two major techniques of Bhakti are: visualization (imagery); repetition of a word or phrase (*japa*).

The visualization takes the form of whatever imagery the devotee finds conducive to arresting and holding his mind. This image is formed internally and if necessary can be reinforced through external representation.

That is, the cherished deity or whatever has been chosen by the devotee as being intensely representative of the principle of Love—any figure, picture, scene that evokes a profound emotional response—is visualized internally as continuously as possible. Amid daily activities the devotee remembers to offer these activities, in an act of self-surrender, to his principle, his image of Love. The reader may question one's ability to retain an image while conducting the everyday business of life, but in a surprisingly short period of practice this becomes entirely possible. The image does not interfere with activity but complements it: as a constant, comforting undertone it lends a new dimension to activity, for now, instead of action bearing the connotation we have previously discussed (desire-action-fulfillment), it becomes, through sacrificial offerings, a medium for self-*dissolution*.

If the internal visualization is weak or if reinforcement is required, the devotee may practice with an "external" aid by placing a replica of the deity, figure, scene, object, etc., before him and reflecting upon it as often as is advisable. The procedure for achieving identification with the essence of the selected replica during concentration is that which has been described in the third through seventh limbs of the Patanjali structure.

The *japa* practice consists of the repetition of a word or phrase. The word or phrase that is given or selected is known as a *mantram* and the repetition of the mantram is japa. Japa may be performed audibly or silently. Again, this is a practice that is performed continuously; the sound is set going and is maintained. There are thousands of traditional mantrams: "Hare Krishna," "Rama, Rama," "Tat twam asi" are some that may be familiar to the reader. Each mantram is the embodiment of a force that has been created by placing certain syllables in particular formations. Through the prescribed rhythm and number of repetitions (japa) the Yogi generates powerful vibrations that activate and free this contained force in a way that enables him to be absorbed in it, and it in him. He effects Yoga (fusion) with it.

Often the visualization and the invocation of the

deity form a simultaneous practice: the Bhakta visualizes the chosen form (internally or externally) and intones a compatible mantram (audibly or silently).

The university students whom we encountered on the campus chanting Sanskrit syllables were intoning a mantram. Some texts treat Mantra as a separate Yoga. The author finds this to be an overly refined distinction. Unless one is utilizing a mantram for personal gain or to achieve some worldly objective, the mantra practice will be performed in that spirit which automatically renders it a practice of Bhakti.

If the reader is attracted to the concept of Bhakti and wishes to undertake its practices he should choose an object of worship in accordance with the principles presented above. This selection is an extremely personal one and we would not influence it other than referring the reader to the above general guidelines. With respect to the choice of a mantram: the Sanskrit phrases and their individual meanings, correct pronunciations, and effective numbers and rhythms of repetition require a much more detailed treatment than can be presented here. However, there is the supreme mantram that can be utilized with great effectiveness by all beings both as a practice in itself and to reinforce any and all imagery. This primary mantram is OM, composed of the three sounds produced by A-U-M.

The eternal cycle of the day and night of Brahma—the cycle of creation, preservation, dissolution, and silence—is represented by A as the first sound (the creation), U as that of preservation, and M, the final sound of dissolution. The actual pronunciation is "Oh-M." Thus, Brahma Itself is the essence of this all-encompassing mantram, the Universal sound. It is the "word" that generates those vibrations which form, sustain, and dissolve all things; OM is the sound that can be heard in the most profound silence. By intoning this supreme mantram the devotee places himself in concordance with the eternal cycle—hence, reidentification, Yoga, through the "word." ("—the Word was with God, and the Word was God.")

The intonation technique is as follows: a deep inhalation is performed slowly. In a low, steady, controlled voice a third of the air in the lungs is used to

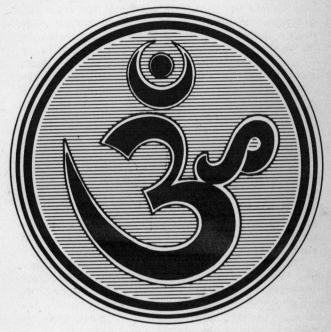

FIG. A — OM—the Primary Mantram

produce the sound "Oh" as if it were coming from the back of the mouth (the lips are shaped in the form of an o); the second third of the air produces the "Oh" sound but it now proceeds from the front of the mouth and is more nasal in character; finally, the lips are pressed together and the remaining third of the air is utilized for the sound of "M." This last should vibrate strongly and the devotee should feel the resonance throughout his head and chest. The mantram is to be intóned as slowly as possible. Begin with approximately ten seconds and, as control is gained, extend the intonation to twenty. When the breath is exhausted pause for several seconds (the pause simulates the "silence" of the cycle, the "withdrawal" of the creation) and begin the next repetition. Perform seven times in a low, steady, controlled voice. Upon completion of the group sit very quietly for as long as is comfortable. Remember that this mantram may be used as a practice in itself or in conjunction with the visualization. Also remember that the Bhakta cultivates his ability to reproduce the mantram *silently* and *continuously*.

With respect to the Patanjali structure, Bhakti Yoga is a development of the second step—the Niyamas—and particularly of the third and fourth qualities: contentment and repeated affirmation of SELF.

Bhakti Yoga, then, is that path which offers reidentification with the Absolute through the quality of Love. It is a path fit for all but is especially suitable for those of intense emotional natures who can recognize the value of directing their feelings into more profound avenues. Its principal techniques are worship and devotion through self-surrender, visualization, and mantra. The reader may undertake to experiment with this Yoga simply by applying the guidelines set forth above.

Chapter 2

Jnana Yoga:
Enlightenment Through Discrimination

Jnana is the path of liberation for those in whom the qualities of the intellect—reason, dialectics, analysis—predominate. The student (Jnani) has gravitated to this Yoga as the result of an intuitive grasp of the fact that he is indeed SELF, that he is always and forever SELF and that he could not for a moment ever be anything but SELF. However, his ordinary mind is still in the dominant position and advances formidable intellectual doubts pertaining to his intuition; he therefore experiences himself as a battleground upon which the forces of intellect and intuition oppose each other. Driven by his intuition to transcend his intellectual doubts he turns to Yoga for guidance and is invited by Jnana to engage in that peculiar and fascinating process wherein *he utilizes ordinary mind to transcend ordinary mind!*

Since the student who is attracted to Jnana generally harbors serious suspicions regarding the omnipotence of ordinary mind, the task of the Guru is to assist him in confirming these suspicions on increasingly deeper levels. Toward this end the student is encouraged to cater to those compelling needs of his ordinary mind—investigation, analysis, evaluation—in conjunction with the application of certain Jnana principles. In this procedure he soon arrives at the point where he recognizes that through his accustomed manner of investigation and analysis he can know only as his ordinary mind and senses permit him to know, that is, in terms of opposites, qualities, distinctions and in a subject-object relationship. He cannot, through ordinary mind, ever know Ultimately and Absolutely. The *intellectual* realization of his inability to Know Absolutely leads the Jnani to aspire, more and more, to that state of consciousness wherein he *shall,* through direct perception, Know Absolutely; wherein he shall, in other words, fuse or effect Yoga with what is to be Known.

The primary principle that is applied by the Jnani to all things is that of *discrimination.* Those propositions that formed the contents of Chapters 1 and 2 in Part I are the very points that comprise the substance of the Jnani's investigations. He examines the nature of maya, of the desire-action-fulfillment pattern, of continually alternating opposites, of the ordinary mind. In all of these he distinguishes his many "I's" in their manifold shapes and forms from the eternal SELF. Through this practice of discrimination, the concealed nature of his ordinary mind and other elements that sustain the illusion of the self are gradually exposed, resulting in the increasing actualization of SELF, that is, in SELF-realization.

As in Bhakti, the practice of Jnana is both active and passive. The principle of discrimination as described above is in effect during all activities, situations, occurrences, encounters. What is Eternal and Real must be distinguished from what is transitory and false—not in dualistic terms of the opposites (good versus bad), but in the absolute sense of SELF. This active discrimination is complemented with passive meditation in which the Jnani may, for example, select an event that has disturbed his equanimity, or consider a "problem" that appears to require resolution. He then examines the elements of this event or problem, not for the purpose of evaluating his actions as right or wrong in the traditional sense of how he determines right and wrong, good and bad, but only with the view toward understanding how the self has prevented or is preventing the SELF from manifesting. The sole "problem" is the obscuration of SELF by self; the Jnani, therefore, seeks to remove the obscuring factors.

There are various applications of the discrimination principle. The great Indian saint of this century, Ramana Maharshi, advocated the highly effective "Who?" inquiry. The student begins by asking "Who am I?" and observes, in as disinterested a manner as possible, the various responses that are presented by his ordinary mind; he will dismiss each response in turn as he realizes that it is only a statistic about a manufactured "self." He continues to inquire "Who am I?" until the ordinary mind has exhausted its responses. Only at this point of exhaustion will he begin to perceive the *true* answer to his question! In Maharshi's teachings the "Who?" technique is to be applied in all situations. For example, when the student finds himself troubled or anxious he is not to examine those elements that he may conjecture are responsible for his difficulty but rather to ask "*Who* is troubled?" or "In *whom* is this anxiety manifesting?" Again, he observes with objectivity the responses that are forthcoming. He perceives that if it is his ordinary mind responding there can be no absolute, real, satisfying answer. Only when his ordinary mind eventually admits that it cannot truly cope with the question will SELF provide the answer that is being sought. This is a process of relentless reintroduction of "illogical input" (the ordinary mind believes that once having furnished a series of statistics it has properly responded to the question; it will regard the continual reintroduction of the identical question as "illogical input"). The student must persist. There is no short-cutting, no circumventing the process of exhausting the ordinary mind's responses. With acute objective attentiveness to all that occurs, the student allows the process to run its full course. The number of days, months, or years that such a course may require will vary in the case of each student and cannot be predetermined; indeed, the serious student always regards the "time" element involved in his practice as totally inconsequential. He practices without anticipation of "progress" because he has begun to perceive the illusionary nature of "progress"; *the practice is its own reward*.

An attendant practice of the Jnani is the study of those scriptures that are concerned with the wisdom and methods of discrimination. The regular readings of such scriptures reinforce the Jnani's resolve to achieve Yoga, point out the multiple deceptions of the ordinary mind and provide techniques to aid in discrimination. For the reader of this book, pertinent Jnanic texts would consist of all *Vedantic* literature, the *Upanishads* (particularly the *Yoga Upanishads*), the *Sutras of Patanjali,* and the recorded words of Ramana Maharshi. (Ramana Maharshi, who was a Guru of the first magnitude, is not to be confused with Maharishi, the "Transcendental Meditation" instructor. We might also note, in passing, that *all* meditation is "transcendental." Excellent English translations are available of these in many public libraries. (See Bibliography.) However, we must caution the student against *excessive* reading. Several paragraphs from any one of the above mentioned works will constitute adequate study on any given day (providing, of course, that each paragraph is reflected upon seriously). Overindulgence in reading and study tends to detract from the essential time that must be devoted to actual *practice*.

The reader who finds himself attracted to the concept of Jnana should regularly read chapters 1 and 2 of Part I. Therein are set forth the principles to be applied in the "active" practice of discrimination. Simultaneously, the techniques described above, or similar techniques of the reader's choosing, should be introduced into his passive meditation practice. Additionally, limited reading and study of the above-indicated works can be included.

Initially, the reader might be led to believe that the Jnana practices would serve to continually reinforce the processes of the ordinary mind rather than to transcend it. But such is not the case. Through the practice of Jnana the ordinary mind is directed into certain channels wherein it is ultimately transformed by that Intelligence of which it is but the palest reflection. The imagery offered in the scriptures to illustrate this process is that of the stick that is used to stir the funeral pyre. In the course of the stirring it eventually ignites and is, itself, consumed.

In the context of the Patanjali structure, Jnana Yoga can be considered as a development of the fifth Niyama: the intellectual resolve to achieve Yoga through discrimination; this is subsequently actualized in the various stages of intuitive knowledge, direct perception, gained in the sixth, seventh, and eighth limbs.

Each system of Yoga contains elements of other Yogas. To be totally involved in Jnana Yoga does not require the elimination of the strong feelings and emotions of Bhakti or preclude use of the physical postures of Hatha. These elements can certainly be included in the Jnani's practice. What *is* implicit in Jnana Yoga is that the practioner, being *primarily* of an intellectual nature, utilizes the principle of discrimination as his major enlightening technique in the attainment of Yoga.

Chapter 3

Karma Yoga:
Inaction in Action

Brahma—God, Supreme Being—is in all things. It is
through Him and only through Him that all things happen, all actions transpire. And yet, being in and acting
through all things He is not *of* them. He is in them and
yet *apart* from them. He is able to initiate action only
because such action is polarized by His principle of
inaction; He is therefore both action in inaction and
inaction in action. He acts and yet does nothing, and it
is only because of Nothingness that Everything occurs!
The ordinary mind evaluates the above as an ultimate
paradox; we have already explained that ordinary mind
is unable to accept that right and wrong, good and
bad, black and white are but alternating manifestations
of a single principle and that these opposites are always and forever inherent in one another. Ordinary
mind will generally have the self identify with whichever end of the stick it presents as desirable or "positive"; the self will then attempt to grasp and make

permanent this aspect, while contriving to hold off the opposite aspect, which it considers "negative" and undesirable. We have seen the futility of these attempts.

When God appears to represent "action" He simultaneously manifests the principle of "inaction." He acts without acting. His action is not concerned with achieving success and avoiding failure. If success were His consideration it would imply that there is some "plan" to be implemented in such a way that it would unfold and conclude successfully. But it is only the ordinary mind that in its conceit and acutely limited perspective demands to "understand" existence by imputing to the creation a "purpose" and then proceeding to question endlessly (and futilely) what this "purpose" might be. *Who* is it that has decided that the creation is purposeful? *Why* must God have a "plan"? What absurd egocentricity the ordinary mind displays in projecting onto the all-encompassing miracle of existence and nonexistence its concepts of "purpose" and "plan"! How bizarre it is to listen to or read the words of those teachers and leaders who would maintain enslavement by explaining God's "plan" for the universe and how this plan is unfolding! As long as one seeks to find the meaning and purpose of life he remains frustrated and ignorant. When the ordinary mind relinquishes such efforts there is no further "problem of man's existence." Meaning and purpose are agonizing fantasies of the ordinary mind. For SELF there are no such fantasies; to be concerned with the "purpose of life" is to sustain ignorance and suffering.

SELF *is*. It has no qualities; it is not tall, short, young, old, intelligent, ignorant, large, small, empty, or full and yet it is simultaneously *all* of these. In Its nothingness it is everything. It does not act and yet it accomplishes all things. The Karma Yogi applies these precepts to his affairs. Karma is not a systemized Yoga, falling into the Patanjali structure or consisting of prescribed practices. It is the emulation on the part of the student of the principle of *inaction in action*. The student is committed to action, but knowing that action performed as part of the desire-action-fulfillment pattern generates new desires that require additional actions, and that this pattern (karma) is eternal, he seeks to act in a way that will terminate, not perpetuate, the pattern. How can this be accomplished?

In chapter 1 we described, at length, the futility of action—regardless of the form it takes—as the means to fulfillment and liberation. And yet all men appear committed to continual action; we have not stated otherwise. What has been implied and what we shall now explicitly state is: The nature of the activity is of small consequence; *the manner in which the action is performed is everything.* SELF acts but does nothing. The student, emulating this principle in order to merge self with SELF, to achieve Yoga, likewise acts, but by divorcing himself from the fruits of his actions, by acting as however he must in all situations, but being *nonattached* to the results—to the success or failure of his actions—breaks the desire-action-fulfillment pattern and is not bound to the consequences of his actions regardless of how these consequences manifest. As such, each action is complete in itself, not a link in a continuing chain or series of actions. To put it another way: all men must act, but the wise man acts dispassionately, in a nonattached manner, without "self" involvement. The actions, then, are no longer *his* actions since they are not performed for self-gratification; he is free of them. The process of karma is thus terminated. In generating no further karma he is subject only to the karma generated by previous actions performed under the direction of the self. When the results, the fruits of these past actions have manifested—be it in this lifetime or, if necessary, additional lifetimes—the cycle of birth and death is concluded. There are no further incarnations for that individual (*jiva*).

The Karma Yoga principle of *inaction in action* is difficult for the novice to grasp. First he equates "inaction" with "doing nothing" and makes the distinction between doing "nothing" and doing "something." But all *doing* is the same. Doing "nothing," which he conceives as passive, is not different than doing "something" in the dynamic sense. All "doing" (action)—from sitting passively and thinking, to dynamic movement—is, in Karma Yoga, equal, equal in the sense that all bears fruit and generates karma. Additionally, as we have seen, no action or series of actions can result in ultimate fulfillment, in achieving Yoga. For the Karma Yogi, then, the art of living lies in his performance of action, the discharging of his duties, *without the intervention of ego, without self-involvement.*

But how can this elusive and alien concept actually be applied to our everyday activities? We have only to conjure up the image of ourselves going through the motions of a typical day to realize how utterly dominant is the ego, the "I," in these events. The technique that is cultivated by the Karma Yogi is the weakening of the ego's hold through the gradual understanding that he is *only an instrument, a vessel through which these events are flowing.* Each time he affirms this truth he causes a disruption in the otherwise continual value judgements imposed by the ordinary mind. Rather than the notion "*I* am experiencing these events," he comes to realize that these events are *flowing through him.* An advanced stage of this realization is reached when the Karma Yogi no longer perceives an event *and* one who is experiencing the event but recognizes that he *is* the event. He thus *becomes his experiences;* the subject-object relationship that has dominated his life dissolves. Outwardly all his activities can appear to go on as before but inwardly a transformation of the first magnitude has occurred: as dominance of the ego, the self, the ordinary mind that constantly reiterates "I am the doer," is diminished and ultimately dissolved, a wonderful sense of freedom results. Rather than a loss of interest or initiative (which one might intellectually suspect would manifest from a nonattachment posture) the Yogi achieves a perspective, balance, and joy in his activities that could not have been experienced previously. This is not the superficial, transitory pleasure that is derived from whatever the self evaluates as "success," but is the *pure* joy that results from no longer having to be concerned with the ordinary mind's concepts of success and failure. Rather than losing interest, initiative, or ability, one's work and activities assume a new dimension of significance that is produced from a *total* rather than a fragmented perspective of action.

It is only when one is able to "let go" of the self,

when it is no longer interjected between the one who acts and the action that results, that SELF-expression (true and original creativity) manifests in his work and action, rather than self-expression (which can only be imitative). All great saints, visionaries, artists, men of letters, composers, and originators in all fields are only too well aware of this fact and they spend a large part of their creative time in developing the technique of transforming the self into an instrument that permits SELF to express its various aspects.

Occupation or religious and philosophical persuasions are of little consequence when one is attracted to the Yoga science. If such occupations or persuasions are to be altered, this will be made known to the student in the course of his practice. It is to be clearly understood that one must never fail to act as he deems necessary and proper in a situation and that he may not interpret the doctrine of nonattachment as license to shirk any responsibility. Discharging all obligations to the best of his ability is an indispensable principle of the Karma Yogi. In so doing, he learns the art of *being in the society but not of the society;* he develops equanimity in all matters and is able to understand various occurrences as the effects of previous actions. He can no longer attribute events to luck, fate, fortune, or accident. The universe is pure Intelligence and he finds himself in harmony with this Intelligence because he is liberated from the "opposites" of the ordinary mind and no longer has any need to perceive the "purpose" of creation. He now accepts everything as it comes, knowing that to rejoice or despair as he has done in the past is to perpetuate his bondage. He understands that through his actions he and he alone—not those convenient phantoms, chance and destiny—is responsible for all that befalls him. His present karma is manifesting because, in the past, he has acted in a particular manner and attached himself to the fruits of these actions. To terminate karma he must divorce himself from his actions, he must apply the principle of nonattachment. Patanjali, in the *Yoga Sutras,* states, "The suffering that has not yet come, *that* is what is to be avoided."

(In these paragraphs we utilize "past," "present,"

and "future" as necessary for explanations and directions. The accomplished Karma Yogi is always aware of "time" as an illusion, as a concept of ordinary mind that is used for convenience on the mayic plane.)

What of morality considerations? If one learns the technique of nonattachment, of acting without generating karma, is he then free to lie, steal, and kill with impunity? The reader might expect an emphatic denial to follow here, but it is not the function of the author to impose the moral judgments dictated by society. We have already listed the five abstentions contained in the Yamas, the first limb of the Patanjali structure. If the beginning student finds such injunctions inadequate to dispel certain strong inclinations he may have in these areas, then he shall have to confront them directly in the context of the application of the Karma Yoga principles. He will then learn, in the most meaningful and profound way, the purpose of these injunctions and how they relate to his development in the practice of Yoga. In the final analysis it is only the student's personal experience, derived from the serious application of the Karma Yoga principles, that can serve as a true code of morality. For the novice to make a prejudgment and characterize the Yogi as "pious" or "puritanical" in the general sense of these words would be to greatly circumscribe his understanding of Yoga. Indeed, for the prospective Yoga student to prejudge the way in which Yogis are "supposed" to think and act is foolish. These things will be KNOWN and manifested *spontaneously* through practice and only through practice. For the student to assume to play the role of a Yogi according to an image he constructs from objective observations or from readings is pointless.

The ordinary mind will eternally regard the doctrines of Karma Yoga as "illogical input" and further elaboration here will serve no purpose. The student must now *experience* what occurs from the application of the "inaction in action" principle; *practice is all*. However, one final paradox should be noted. In the course of his practice, the Karma Yogi must be nonattached to nonattachment. That is, if nonattachment becomes a constant objective, an obsession, it is always present as an unfulfilled desire. This would be contrary to our intention. Therefore, equanimity must also be maintained in the cultivation of nonattachment, and while no formula or direction can be offered for this purpose it is our experience that the student soon discerns the delicate balance point: he learns how to lean but not push, how to back off without relinquishing responsibility, how to remain aware without judging. In short, what is initially the *desire* to become nonattached to one's actions is, in the actual practice, divested of its "desire" dynamics and transformed into a selfless, nongrasping way of life.

The principles of Karma Yoga are basic to all Yogas and are applied in conjunction with whatever system occupies the student's primary interest. The previously mentioned "business executive" who informs us that in the course of his daily business activities he is applying the principles of Yoga has reference to Karma Yoga. He is practicing to achieve "inaction in action."

The reader is urged to obtain a copy of the *Bhagavad Gita*, a sublime presentation of the doctrine of Karma Yoga that is the most widely read and studied scriptural work in India.

> One of dull intellect, even
> without doing anything is ever
> agitated by distraction; but the
> skillful one, even doing his duties
> is verily unperturbed.
> —Astavakra Samhita

Chapter 4

Raja Yoga:
Reintegration in Stillness

In the classical texts, Raja Yoga is described as the "Royal Path," or the "Yoga of Light" ("raja" meaning "radiance"). It is said that this Yoga holds the key to the *final* step, to the *ultimate* state. Just as Karma Yoga must be practiced in conjunction with all other Yogas, so will all students eventually reach that point in their practice where they require the vehicle of Raja to be carried "on the final journey to the other shore."

Raja Yoga is synonymous with the Patanjali structure; it parallels the eight steps or limbs that we have learned. But whereas in our previous outline of the structure we have listed the eighth step, Samadhi, simply as the final limb, as the ultimate objective of Yoga practice, we must now note that *there are a series of gradations in Samadhi*. Although to the beginning student a description of these fine gradations is unintelligible it is necessary to know, at least intellectually, that they are the essence of Raja Yoga. The significance of Raja is this: when the student achieves his initial objective in Samadhi and uncovers the SELF, he is to understand that he is experiencing only an *aspect* of SELF and that his absorption, his Yoga, is still incomplete. He *must* be aware of this incompleteness because these initial experiences of SELF are so overwhelming, resulting in such an intense joy that he is inclined to believe the final objective has been attained. But the Raja principle of "netti, netti" ("not this, not this is yet the ultimate goal") enjoins him to press on to the next stage, and then to the next. Regardless of what power, knowledge, or ecstasy is experienced at each succeeding stage of Samadhi the student must not luxuriate in it but continue his meditation practice until the ultimate state is reached.

Patanjali defines the objective of Yoga as "the restraint of mental modifications," that is, the unqualified quieting of the ordinary mind. The words "restraint" and "quieting" in this context are synonymous with "silence," "stillness," "emptiness." We have noted that the various Yoga techniques previously described have the objective of first arresting, eventually quieting, and ultimately transcending the ordinary mind. For example, in the intoning of a mantram (audibly or silently) we seek to fix our attentions on the *sound* and, by so doing, interrupt the process of incessant "thinking." Although in initial attempts the attention is frequently distracted (this "wavering attention" is designated as Dharana, the sixth step of the Patanjali structure), with continued serious practice that includes acute concentration on the words and not simply their unconscious repetition, the *principal vibration* or *essence* of the mantram begins to penetrate the consciousness. At this stage the ordinary mind becomes less and less distracted because it is held increasingly transfixed by the sound vibration. (This "steady" concentration is Dhyana, the seventh step.) Eventually, the vibration of the mantram awakens the sympathetic vibration of SELF. When this occurs, SELF emerges, and ordinary mind assumes its natural, subservient role; it is greatly weakened in its ability to divert; now it is "restrained" and the eighth limb, Samadhi, is attained. But the Yoga is incomplete: while having made contact with SELF, self's absorption (Yoga) into SELF may be but momentary and oblique, for ordinary mind cannot be long quieted; its motions resume, it disassociates from SELF, it reestablishes self-identity, it reasserts its dominant role, and SELF is once again obscured.

Therefore, the objective of practice at this stage becomes the extending of the period of contact and absorption. Toward this end the Yogi may continue to utilize his mantram (or whatever his primary technique is). The practice should be maintained during his everyday activities, but the major developments will occur during his passive periods of meditation. During each absorption in SELF, self is transformed so that upon its disassociation it comes away with more attributes and qualities of SELF. The point is reached where SELF can be readily contacted; now the vehicle for contact (mantram, visualization, pranayama, etc.) may be abandoned; it has served its purpose and is no longer required.

The subtle "stages" of transformation that self experiences in its contact with SELF were known to the ancient seers to the extent that each such stage was named according to its characteristics. A description of these stages would be superfluous here; indeed, it may never be necessary for even the serious student to learn their names and characteristics in an academic context. Dedicated practice and internal instruction can divulge all that one must Know. But even in these advanced stages of Samadhi the Yoga is designated as "incomplete." The reason for this is that although self's absorption in, and transformation through, SELF continues to increase, there remains the separate and distinct awareness of SELF by self. Even when deeply immersed in SELF, there is still "self" awareness. In other words, the Yoga is not final as long as a separation in the form of awareness or recognition of SELF by self remains. This separation, however subtle, is distinguished in Raja Yoga from an *ultimate unification* wherein there is no longer any awareness of a separation and wherein the mergence, or Yoga, is complete. The former is designated as *samprajnata* Samadhi and denotes *conscious knowledge* or awareness of self's identification with SELF; the latter is designated as *asamprajnata* Samadhi and denotes identification *with-*

out individual, conscious knowledge. In asamprajnata the self's absorption is complete; it has taken the final step on the path and has returned permanently to its original abode, SELF. The final Yoga is achieved; the manifold illusions of maya cannot reappear.

The ordinary mind is instantaneously filled with a multitude of pressing questions about this "final" re-integration. "What happens there? Does one continue to 'live' in the physical sense? Does he function as an 'ordinary' person?" But asamprajnata Samadhi is *pure experience.* The ordinary mind cannot experience, it can only evaluate mayic statistics. Since advanced Samadhi represents ultimate transcendence of ordinary mind, how can ordinary mind comprehend what is involved when it has been totally transcended? Speculation in such transcendental matters by the ordinary mind will only divert valuable time and energy from practice. Consequently, we shall here pull the ordinary mind up short by stating that all things pertaining to Samadhi will, in due course, be Known to the student through his dedicated practice. Of this there is not the slightest doubt.

Some additional guidance in the actual practice of passive meditation, directed to the beginning-intermediate student, should prove helpful. With respect to the Patanjali structure (which we have noted is synonymous with Raja Yoga), this guidance is concerned with steps five, six, and seven. Steps three and four—Asana and Pranayama—will be treated in Part III. Step eight—Samadhi—will not concern the student at present. Steps one and two have been presented in detail.

Having entered into that quiet, peaceful area that he reserves for his concentration-meditation practice, and having assumed the proper seated position and regulated his breathing (as described in Part III), the student contacts his senses—primarily those of sight and sound—and withdraws them from external stimuli. (This is step five, Pratyahara, the conscious withdrawal and deactivation of the senses.) Then, selecting the element, object, or thought for his "seed" of concentration, he proceeds to fix his consciousness as fully and as steadily as possible upon this seed. Although his resolve to concentrate is firm, it is not obsessive; no tension should be experienced. At first, it may be difficult to maintain the required concentration for more than a few seconds in each attempt during the practice session. That is, having resolved to fix his attention on a particular point, the student, nonetheless, is beset by an onslaught of thoughts that act to distract his attention. He may spend a surprising amount of time involved in these thoughts and be unaware that such is the case! So he must be alert to the arising of distractions. He never becomes impatient or angry; he simply dismisses the thoughts or distracting stimuli as quickly as he becomes aware of them and returns his attention to his "seed." This sixth step, in which the attention is prone to wander, is Dharana.

With regular, serious concentration sessions the student gains facility in the practice, and the intervals of fixation are extended to several minutes without interruption. At this point Dharana becomes Dhyana, the seventh limb, uninterrupted fixation. It is here that the student begins to Know the meaning and effects of concentration; it is in Dhyana that he gains the deeper "sense" and "feeling" of Yoga. The necessary procedure beyond this point, into Samadhi, will certainly be revealed to the student when he is ready. This is as inevitable as any organic process of which the reader is aware.

What is the frequency and length of practice sessions? The student's significant development will be dependent on regular practice: once or twice daily, at the same hour (preferably upon arising and again at sundown or shortly before retiring). One may begin with as little as a five-minute interval and gradually extend it to as long as is comfortable and practical. Advanced students will often spend an hour or more in each session. When the legs tire in the seated position they may be reversed or extended outward with as little movement and disturbance as possible and the session continued in one of these altered positions. The ability to sit with comfort in the various seated positions increases quickly with practice. It is also feasible to divide the session into two segments, with several minutes of Hatha Yoga asanas being performed between the segments.

In the beginning phase the ordinary mind will present every possible excuse—from the most subtle to the most overt—to prevent the student from undertaking regular concentration practice. The ordinary mind recognizes the great threat to its position that is inherent in this practice and will utilize all of its resources in diverting the student from it. As the time for practice draws near the most insignificant activity that may delay or cancel the session will suddenly assume the greatest urgency in the student's ordinary mind. But if he can overcome these devices of the ordinary mind and persevere in his regular sessions for a period of several months he will no longer be dissuaded because at that point the situation is reversed: *nothing assumes greater importance than his Yoga practice.*

The student does not look for "results" from his practice. For many months he will be in no position to evaluate his "progress" and he must make no attempt to do so. He simply continues his serious, patient, and regular practice with nonattachment; his only objective is to steady his attention and quiet his mind. Then there comes a time when he is suddenly very much aware of the profound development that has been occurring all the while! From this point on he requires no further incentive; he now Knows that his fulfillment and peace lie in the "stillness" within, and that the eight steps of Yoga comprise a path to that stillness.

Chapter 5

Laya Yoga:
Man as the Universe

All that is contained in the Creation, from its most subtle planes (the innumerable "heaven worlds" of Asian theology) to the gross universe that is perceived by the five senses, is also present in man. When the creation is actualized, man is simultaneously actualized.

The ordinary mind, in its endless and futile speculations as to its own origins, has relatively recently developed a theory of man's "evolution." This new ingredient of the mayic conspiracy, currently accepted by a large segment of the world's population, postulates that man has *reached* (evolved into) his present state of advanced (but imperfect) development through a series of transformations: microbe, fish, and ape are some of the stops along the way. In the context of Yoga this theory cannot claim our attention for more than a moment. Man, a projection of Brahma, "made in the image of God," has never been other than Complete and Perfect. But few truths are less acceptable to the ordinary mind of Western man. How can it (ordinary mind) engage in its cherished activity of "self-improvement," on which it thrives, if Perfection already IS? No, it will have none of this illogical "Perfection" input. Left to its own devices, ordinary mind will make certain that civilized man will spend all eternity becoming a "better" creature by "discovering" his potential, "expanding" his consciousness, and through other, innumerable self-improvement ventures to which we have previously alluded. At the same time, ordinary mind makes it clear that man can never actually *arrive* at the ultimate state of Perfection (an important axiom of the conspiracy is that "nobody's perfect"), but he can *become* an increasingly improved person. He may *approach* God in an eternal subject-object relationship but he can surely never *become* perfect enough to BE ONE WITH God.

In Reality, man *never becomes* SELF; he IS SELF. Man *never grows or evolves* into Completeness and Perfection; he is NOW these things. Ordinary mind first conceives "perfection-imperfection" and then proceeds to find imperfection wherever it pleases. In short, ordinary mind, ego, is itself the principle and instrument of imperfection and it knows this imperfection by virtue of its opposite, perfection. There is no imperfection apart from self. Man is NOW Complete and Perfect and could not be otherwise. The transcendence of self, so that SELF, the true state of Perfection may be recognized, is the objective of Yoga practice.

The universe (*all* aspects of creation) exists on many levels simultaneously. Man exists in this identical simultaneity; he is a complex of dimensions. Western psychologists indicate some knowledge of this complex with their terms "conscious," "subconscious," and "unconscious." Man can KNOW these dimensions as he journeys on a particular path to achieving Yoga. Laya Yoga is the system that is concerned with this path.

In describing the process of creation the texts of Laya Yoga symbolically designate the ONE, the ALL, the UNDIVIDED as the deity Shiva. In the act of creation, Shiva, willing that the ONE shall become many, causes a vibration. From this vibration there issues forth a *projection* of Shiva in the form of a force, known in

78

Sanskrit as a *shakti* (power), that becomes Shiva's agent in implementing the creation. The *shakti*, carrying with it all aspects of Shiva, manifests these aspects, with their multitudinous forms and species of life, in a series of dimensions or planes (*lokas*). These planes are distinguished from one another primarily by the elements of which they are composed; they range in order from those that are of the most ethereal and subtle forms to those of the most gross and dense matter. In essence, the creation manifests in *increasing degrees of density* wherein spirit—Brahma, Shiva, God—becomes embodied in denser and denser matter. This process culminates in the formation of the physical universe, composed of extremely dense matter.

The creation manifests simultaneously as the *macrocosm* (universe) and the *microcosm* (man). Man is connected to each plane of the creation, and vice versa, through a specific area of his organism: the brain, throat, heart, and navel are some of the major areas involved. Each of these areas—representing a dimension of the creation—has its focal point or control plexus within what we know, anatomically, as the "spine." The following is a description of the creation as it manifests microcosmically, according to the Laya Yoga shastras.

The abode of Shiva is in the area just above the top of the skull, actually *external* to the physical sheath. The shakti, in issuing forth from Shiva and proceeding to manifest the creation, moves through the head and then, in a descending direction, within what is eventually to be designated as "the hollow of the central canal of the spine." There are five major points along this canal where *centers* or focal points are established by the shakti. Each of these centers relates to an area of the body which, in turn, corresponds to a particular dimension of the creation. These dimensions (as the shakti descends) are composed of increasingly gross elements. When the final of these centers is established in the area at the base of the spine, the physical body has been formed and the work of the shakti is complete. The *cosmic* axis is thus duplicated as the *spinal* axis. When we write that the shakti "descends within the spine," it must be understood that the spine does not exist in its final *physical* form until the creation is completed. The organism is being formed and the centers are being established simultaneously. *The "canal" that contains the centers is actually situated within the subtle, ethereal bodies or sheaths around which the physical spine is formed.*

In all this Shiva Itself does nothing; It remains always the *passive* principle. Its agent, shakti, a projection of Itself which it invests with all of Its aspects and the power to manifest these aspects, is the *dynamic* principle. However, having once completed its work with the formation of the physical sheath, the shakti is rendered inactive. It then sleeps in a dormant, static, but *potentially dynamic* state at the base of the spine. Because of the way in which the shakti rests coiled, in a serpentine manner, at the base of the spine it is designated as the *Kundalini shakti (kundala = coil).*

The ordinary man, living primarily in his physical body, perceiving a gross world through his five senses and imprisoned in the mayic structure by his ordinary mind, is largely unaware of the other planes of his existence, unaware that he is Brahma cloaked in a complex of sheaths. The practitioners of Laya Yoga attribute this ignorance to the sleeping of kundalini: having manifested a particular aspect or plane of the creation —of which the corresponding "center" in the spine is the focal point—the kundalini shakti leaves this center to continue its descending journey. It is the dynamic *presence* of kundalini that energizes and activates the center and thus makes it a reality to the consciousness. Without this dynamicism the center is greatly diminished in its vitality and functions falteringly since it can draw only on the original energy that was deposited by kundalini. Because, in the ordinary man, the kundalini lies sleeping, he has little conscious awareness of the centers.

Laya means "absorption." The objective of Laya Yoga is to reawaken the kundalini and to lead it through the six major centers (five within the spine and one in the area between the eyebrows). When, through the prescribed practices, the kundalini *is* awakened it "pierces" the centers in an ascending order, beginning with the lowest, the Muladhara. As it dwells in any particular center, that center is revitalized and the plane of existence of which it is the essence becomes KNOWN. The implications of "known" are that the individual can function among and even control the elements of which that particular plane is composed. It is through this process that many of the so-called "powers" (*siddhis*) of the Yogi are gained. But here again, whatever power or knowledge is derived from any given plane will be acknowledged in a disinterested manner by the true Yogi, for to become involved with these things is to seriously curtail his journey. So while he achieves Yoga with a particular plane, to realize his final objective he must move on. He absorbs (*laya*) the essence of that plane and practices to lead kundalini upward to the next center. As kundalini leaves a center, continuing its ascending journey, it carries with it the essence of that center (and of all preceding centers through which it has passed). That center is then rendered inactive; it ceases to function altogether. The ultimate objective is to direct kundalini back to its place of origin—to the abode of Shiva whence it issued forth. There, returning with its bountiful harvest that it has absorbed from the six centers, the kundalini shakti is reunited with its source. The resultant Yoga is described by those who practice Laya as a "cosmic intercourse."

During this experience the consciousness reposes outside of the physical organism (above the physical skull); certain vital functions of the organism are suspended and the body grows cold except for heat that continues to radiate from the top of the skull. When kundalini separates from Shiva and returns to the organism the exact reverse process occurs: kundalini redeposits, with increased prana, those elements that were absorbed in its ascension, so that following each descent the centers function with much greater vitality. This results in the student's increasing awareness of the various dimensions of the creation, not only during his meditation practice but amid all activities of his everyday life.

How many centers are "pierced" during any single ascent of kundalini and how long kundalini remains in each will vary with the practitioner and is dependent upon the type and intensity of practice. The Laya Yogi gains increasing facility in directing kundalini and eventually arrives at the point where, having reunited kundalini with Shiva, he may choose to retain this ultimate Yoga and not return kundalini to the organism. The determining factors of this choice are highly subjective and it would be premature to consider them here.

There are six major centers. Each has certain distinguishing characteristics; it is the knowledge of such characteristics and the prescribed application of this knowledge that are instrumental in preparing that center for activation. The pertinent characteristics include: geometric form, dominant color, inherent sound, type of power, and controlling deity. The geometric forms and the colors of the centers are universal. That is, wherever in the world a man would be conscious of the opening of a center, he would perceive the approximate form and color in that center that is described in the treatises pertaining to Laya Yoga. But other characteristics indicated in these texts—such as the deities and sounds—seem to be superimposed on the centers and are Indian in character. If the reader is attracted to the concept of Laya his two major considerations for the present should be (1) locations of the centers; (2) cultivation of the ability to visualize their principal forms. These two points become the bases of actual practice in part III.

We have stated that the centers are located in the subtle (ethereal) sheaths, not in the physical body. Consequently, they are not visible to the physical eye. But any particular center *can* be seen through the internal vision when that center has been activated and the consciousness dwells there. The geometric form of each center appears to be contained within a circle and consequently the centers are designated in the pertinent texts as *chakras,* Sanskrit for "circles" or "wheels." The chakras (situated in the subtle sheaths) are connected to their corresponding spheres of influence in the gross, physical body through an extensive network of subtle channels. These channels (*nadis*) are not physical veins, arteries, or nerves, but subtle conduits through which *prana*, energy, is conveyed from the centers to the physical body. It is this prana that is responsible for maintaining the "life" of the physical body. The manner in which the nadis join at the various centers creates the appearance of lotuses with petals. The Laya Yoga texts, in describing the chakras, include information as to the number of petals (ranging from two to sixteen) of each.

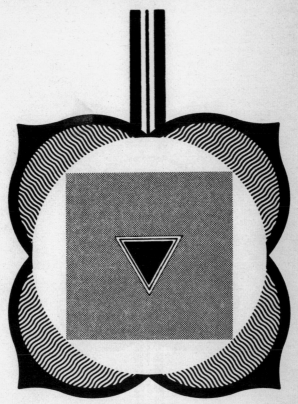

FIG. B — Muladhara Chakra

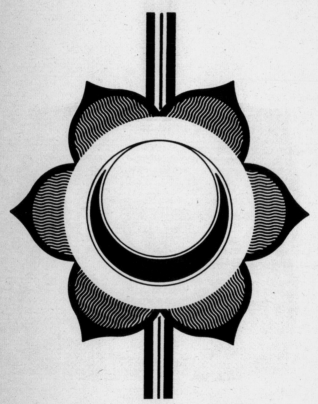

FIG. C — Savadhishthana Chakra

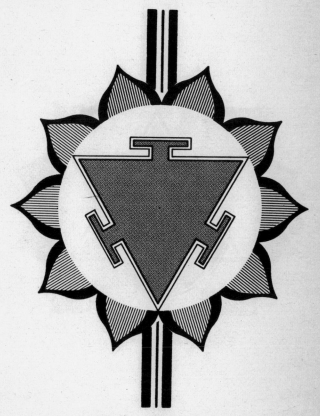

FIG. D — Manipura Chakra

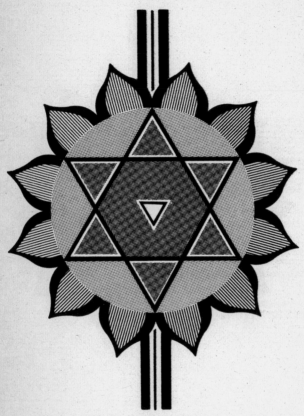

FIG. E — Anahata Chakra

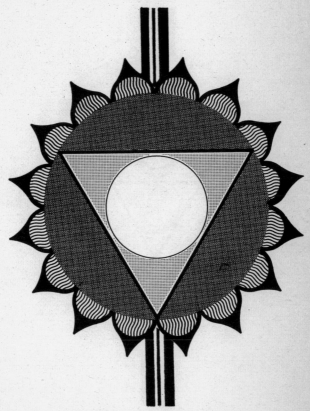

FIG. F — Vishuddha Chakra

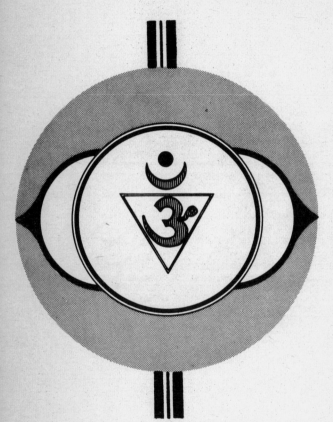

FIG. G—Ajna Chakra

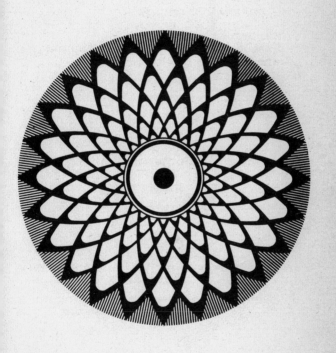

FIG. H — Sahasrara

	CHAKRA	LOCATION	PRINCIPAL FORM
	Sahasrara— the abode of Shiva	Above the physical skull	Thousand-petal Lotus
6.	Ajna	Between the eyebrows	Circle
5.	Vishuddha	Throat	Circle within inverted triangle
4.	Anahata	To the right of the physical heart	Hexagon within circle
3.	Manipura	Navel	Triangle (inverted) within circle
2.	Savadhishthana	At the root of the genitals	Crescent within circle
1.	Muladhara	Midway between the anus and the genitals	Triangle within square

FIG. I — Description of the Chakras

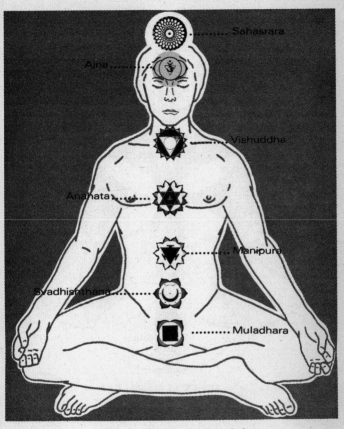

FIG. J — Position of the Chakras

91

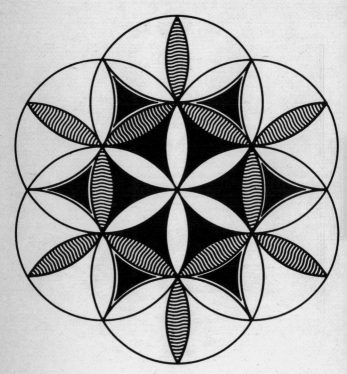

FIG. K — Yantra

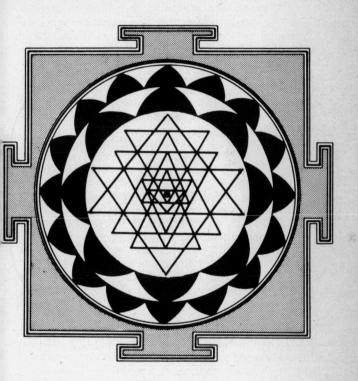

FIG. L — Yantra

The kundalini is aroused through both meditative and physiological practices. The physiological techniques include *asana, pranayama, mudra*—all to be treated in Part III. The meditative practices include *mantra* and *yantra*. We have described *mantra* in chapter 5. A *yantra* is a geometric form that becomes a "seed" for concentration. Just as a mantram embodies a vibration or force which through repetition (japa) with acute awareness eventually awakens and unites with the sympathetic vibration of SELF, so does a yantra embody a similar vibration. The yantric force is contained within a symmetric design. There are a multitude of traditional yantras that are of varying degrees of complexity and that represent different aspects of the creation.

Students who wish to prepare for the activation of the chakras, while simultaneously developing their abilities to concentrate, will find the appropriate method for yantra visualization in part III. In addition to the chakra yantras, other important yantras are included there. (Certain elaborations upon yantras are known as *mandalas;* these will not concern us in this book.)

The numerous subjective experiences inherent in Laya Yoga cannot receive comprehensive treatment in written form. As in all Yogas, the experiences defy description. The purpose of this chapter is to acquaint the reader with the existence of the chakras and the bodies, both physical and subtle, as the microcosmic manifestation of creation, and to indicate that the practices contained in part III may be undertaken by him to prepare the centers for the awakening of kundalini. This preparation must take the forms of a thorough purification and strengthening of the entire organism; unless this is accomplished the kundalini cannot be safely aroused. Should it be forced or otherwise prematurely aroused the consequences can be dangerous. Therefore, in Part III the preparatory practices are described but not the techniques for the direct, conscious stimulation of the kundalini. The student interested in Laya should focus his full attention on the preparatory practices. When he has perfected these he may refer to the definitive English-language treatise on Kundalini Yoga: *The Serpent Power,* by Sir John Woodroffe.

There are a number of *mystical* or highly esoteric approaches to Yoga that are classified as "Tantric." Laya is designated as one of these.

PART III

The Body as a Path to Self

*Hatha Yoga is a refuge for all those
who are scorched by the fires. To those
who practice Yoga, Hatha Yoga is
like the tortoise that supports the world.*

—Hatha Yoga Pradipika

Chapter 1

Hatha Yoga:
The Theory

(1)

Hatha Yoga is described as "that system which renders the consciousness fit for concentration."

Although in the *Sutras* Patanjali uses only the *word*
"asana" without elaborating on the technique involved,
it is probable that, since asana means "steady and comfortable posture," he refers to those seated, folded-leg
positions which we know as the "Lotus" postures and
which enable the Yogi to properly accommodate his
body for the intervals of time necessary in the practice of
pranayama and the four succeeding steps of the structure. In the more advanced concentration-meditation
practices, the body must remain quiet and steady for
lengthy intervals. When perfected, the Half- and Full-
Lotus postures, common in India since time immemorial, offer the most satisfactory solution to protracted
sitting, since they provide both "steadiness" and "comfort." Also, there are attendant techniques applied by

the Yogi that render the Lotus postures fit to function as actual *aids* in meditation.

In most systems of Yoga the Lotus postures are the only asanas necessary. But in Hatha Yoga, asana, the third limb, is comprised of an extensive series of poses other than seated ones. Pranayama, breath regulation, the fourth limb, only alluded to by Patanjali and utilized minimally in other Yogas, becomes in Hatha a detailed science. How many such asanas or breath-control techniques (*kumbhakas*) were known and applied prior to Patanjali we cannot say with accuracy, but it is probable that the basic form in which Hatha Yoga is now practiced was developed during the ten centuries following Patanjali, with periodic modifications since the Middle Ages.

Let us enumerate the primary objectives of Hatha Yoga:

1. *Cultivate a high level of health and promote longevity*

   a. Foster endurance, strength, muscle tone, vitality, flexibility, good circulation, weight control

   b. Eliminate toxic and debilitating conditions through purification of the organism

2. *Stabilize and quiet the ordinary mind*

   a. Develop the ability to concentrate
      (1) Fixation of the consciousness on the asana movements
      (2) Visualization as instructed

   b. Apply those techniques that are specifically designed for sense relaxation and withdrawal
      (1) Control and transformation of energies
      (2) Control and suspension of breath

3. *Awaken the kundalini*

We will next examine these objectives in greater detail.

1. Cultivate a high level of health and promote longevity

a. The Hatha Yoga techniques recondition and develop every area of the physical organism. They accomplish these with great ingenuity and effectiveness and it is only necessary for the student to undertake the Hatha program with dedication in order to experience the health benefits that are inherent therein. The value of endurance, vitality, controlled weight, etc., and the resultant possibility of longevity without illness is obvious. I have written extensively on these matters and refer the interested reader to the pertinent books (see Bibliography).

It is the "health" aspect of Hatha Yoga that has been its major attraction for the Western world; the current interest in health enables many "teachers" who have very little knowledge of the more profound objectives of Hatha (or Yoga in general) to be able to fill their classes on a continuing basis. The asanas are so effective that even when they are taught in what is only a partially competent manner there can be dramatic results. The current "demand" for Hatha instruction has created a multitude of "teachers" who are entirely untrained in Yoga; gym teachers, dance instructors, or just those who have become proficient in the asanas are now "instructing." The tragedy of this is that the "health" aspect continues to be emphasized as the principal merit of Hatha and students who emerge from the classes taught by untrained "teachers" continue to believe that Yoga is a practice that is primarily concerned with relaxation, weight control, and flexibility. The smattering of chanting and homespun philosophy that may be offered in these classes usually has little to do with Yoga. If there is concentration-meditation practice it is generally unproductive, since the genuine attainments of the "teachers" who are conducting such meditation are extremely limited and what we have is a classic example of "the blind leading the blind." One simply cannot teach what one does not know.

Each day the author receives letters from persons connected with schools and recreational organizations of every imaginable type who state that they are about to initiate Yoga courses in their respective institutions and can information be sent as to how to proceed? What has occurred is that the deans or directors have contacted them, indicated that there seems to be community interest in Yoga, and asked that they organize Yoga classes. They are therefore requesting literature that they can peruse for several days or weeks that will render them fit and qualified to instruct Yoga. Were these people to offer a course in English Literature or in the History of Ancient Greece it would undoubtedly be necessary for them to be thoroughly knowledgeable not only in the subject matter but in the pertinent teaching techniques. Even a meaningful course in Volleyball would necessitate more than cursory preparation. But, acting on their own impulses or those of the aforesaid officials, most seem ready and willing to instruct Hatha Yoga (a subject requiring many years of the most serious study and practice) with little more knowledge than what has been gleaned from a book or two and a few words of advice and encouragement from the author!

In the serious practice of Hatha, a high level of health and an unparalleled sense of well-being *should* be experienced. This is the "Health" of our "Eight Steps to Health and Peace." And it is true that, initially, the student may be attracted to a Yoga class by the "health" aspect. But very early on in this class *he must be informed that "health" represents only a fragment of the system*. In certain texts a warning is cited on the "danger" of Hatha practice. I interpret this "danger" to the student in terms of his undertaking the study solely on the *physical* level—becoming preoccupied with his health and physical appearance—and thereby remaining ignorant of both the practice and *total experience* of Hatha. The "teacher" who is attempting to instruct Hatha on the basis of physical fitness—with a dash of Westernized emotional and mental health tossed in—does a great disservice to himself and to his students. All readers who consider attending a Hatha Yoga class should carefully evaluate the instructor in terms of what has been stated above.

b. "Purification" pertains to the general hygiene, cleansing, nutrition, and fasting practices which have been alluded to in this book and which I have described in detail in other writings. In addition to the above, purification is accomplished through pranayama and those asanas that aid in breaking down deposits and improving circulation and elimination.

2. Stabilize and quiet the ordinary mind

Here we can begin to appreciate the true profundity of Hatha Yoga. In a *physiological* approach, the body becomes the instrument through which the ordinary mind may be quieted and SELF recognized!

a. With respect to the asanas the mind-stabilization process is an active-passive one: the body of the student is active in that it moves in and out of the positions while his mind is involved in the movements in such a way that the entire organism eventually becomes *the vehicle through which the movements flow.* Self is absorbed in the movements of SELF.

The passive aspect of the process relates to *visualization.* Once the extreme position of the pose is assumed it is *held motionless.* The word "asana" actually denotes this static position. The consciousness is then directed either to the physical area which is being emphasized in the extreme position or it is occupied with the visualization of certain yantras. Either of these may be utilized as the "seed" for concentration, for the fixation of ordinary mind.

b. In addition to the naturally quieting properties of the asana itself, there are certain techniques such as the placing of pressure on critical points, the control and redirecting of the flow of energies, and the suspension of breath that drive the consciousness inward.

3. Awaken the kundalini

The Hatha Yoga course presented in chapter 2 will prepare the student to awaken and raise the kundalini. However, because the actual arousal of kundalini is highly complex and involves extremely advanced practices which will require some time for the student to thoroughly master, we shall not advocate application of any of the techniques described in this book specifically toward that end.

The Hatha Yoga shastras present the following cosmological description of the inception of the asanas: *Through a type of cosmic "dance" an agent of Shiva revealed 8,400,000 bodily positions to mankind. Of these, eighty-four are fit for the practicing Yogi of this yuga (age).* Of these eighty-four, we find approximately forty to be highly effective and practical for regular practice.

The asanas lend themselves to various classifications: static-dynamic, active-passive, convex-concave, extension-retraction. The physiological implications of these should be known to all Hatha *instructors*. But here we are primarily concerned with encouraging the reader to become involved in the serious practice of one or more of the Yogas, among which Hatha should be included. For this purpose, only specific knowledge for correct execution of the asanas is necessary.

The asanas are performed in an extremely elementary, nonstrenuous manner by the beginning student. In gradual stages, without regard for the "time" involved, the student gains aptitude and proceeds to the intermediate and eventually more advanced stages of the asanas. In our method most of the asanas are performed in slow motion with a "holding" interval in the extreme position.

We have defined "asana" as "steady and comfortable position," and have noted that the word originally designated one of the passive, seated, folded-leg postures. Eventually, "asanas" came to denote not only these seated postures but an extensive series of varied poses that are held in a static, frozen, motionless manner. Ultimately, the definition was extended to include the movements that led into and out of these poses, each pose being regarded as the "extreme position" of a particular series of movements. "Steady and comfortable" implies that the series of movements are performed, and the extreme position maintained, with "ease." Such ease is accomplished, of course, with practice; the student practices seriously, regularly, and patiently and may be obliged to experience certain periods of minor discomfort (never *strain*) to eventually arrive at the "comfortable" stage. The well-known concert artist, previously mentioned, who is depicted in the Head Stand may have reached this stage of "ease"; he finds the inverted posture not only relaxing and revitalizing but highly conducive to concentration!

Being able to maintain the extreme position with ease for longer intervals is important because the general benefits to be derived from that position are then increased. Strength and endurance result and, most important, the ability to steady the mind and achieve one-pointedness is developed. In each of the extreme positions the consciousness is fixed and remains upon a given point. But there is an extraordinary interaction here: while the consciousness is being directed to the indicated point the regulation of breath, coupled with the configuration of the body in that extreme position, attracts and holds the consciousness. This, then, is one of the most profound aspects of Hatha Yoga: *it is the asana itself that acts to steady and ultimately transcend the ordinary mind.*

In the elementary stages of practice the student is directed to fix his attention on that area of the body which is involved in the extreme position of a particular asana—where he experiences the stress or emphasis. If the lumbar area of the back is being stretched, *that* is the area for him to "feel," to which he must direct his undivided attention. It should be noted that the physical or therapeutic value of the asana is also increased through this "feeling" technique. In the more advanced stages, when the student has developed his ability to steady the mind and is beginning to experience Hatha Yoga as a more spiritual and less physical practice, he can undertake the visualization of the *yantras.* Complete instructions for both of these concentration practices, as well as for the execution of the asanas, are presented in the text of chapter 2.

Pranayama, the fourth step of the Patanjali structure, designates a system of *breath-control and regulation* exercises. We have learned that to successfully accomplish the objectives of concentration it is necessary that the ordinary mind be steadily fixed upon one point and eventually stilled. In this regard pranayama plays an indispensable role; its practice is utilized in various forms in all systems of Yoga where concentration-meditation is indicated.

As the breath moves, so moves the mind. If breathing is irregular, erratic, obstructed, the mind is correspondingly disturbed; if breathing is rhythmic, quiet, and unobstructed the mind can become tranquil and steady. When respiration can be regulated to the degree that it is slowed in the extreme, the thoughts subside to a corresponding degree. It then follows that if respiration is *suspended,* thoughts will be likewise suspended. If the reader, at this very moment, will make a conscious effort to slow and quiet his breathing—simply by fixing his attention on it—he will note that his mind begins to relax accordingly.

The word "pranayama" is a combination of "prana" (defined in this context as "breathing") and "ayama" ("pause"). Thus "pranayama" would translate as "breathing that is lengthened by a pause." The pause denotes an interruption in the process of respiration by an *intentional suspension* (*kumbhaka*) that is imposed at the end of a measured inhalation (*puraka*) or at the end of a measured exhalation (*rechaka*). (Additionally, there is a technique of suspension that is applied at any point during respiration; i.e., the advanced Yogi cultivates the ability to suspend his breathing at any point during an inhalation or exhalation. This is designated as *kevala kumbhaka*.) We are, then, involved with three elements: inhalation, exhalation, and suspension. Variations in the action and rhythm of these comprise the science of pranayama. (In the classical texts, "pranayama" frequently becomes synonymous with the word "kumbhaka" because most of the breathing exercises of the system contain one or more suspensions, and it is these suspensions that are of paramount importance in achieving the Hatha Yoga objectives.)

In chapter 5, "Laya Yoga," we noted the existence of the *nadis,* a network of conduits in the subtle body through which life-force is conducted to the gross physical body. Through the respiration process, gross elements such as oxygen and carbon are absorbed directly by the physical body but the subtle element, prana, the force or essence that actually sustains life, is collected by the subtle body and channeled into the physical body. It is intended that the prana should flow freely through the nadis so as to maintain a high level of health of the physical body; health is said to be impaired to the extent that the nadis are obstructed by deposits, sediments, and various impurities accumulated by the physical organism. Ultimately, these impurities have a congesting effect on the nadis. But apart from the health aspect there are the essential esoteric objectives that cannot be realized as long as such congestion exists. Consequently, Hatha Yoga includes a number of intensive *cleansing* practices that are basic to the course. Asana and pranayama are, in themselves, "acts of purification." They break down deposits, promote good circulation to improve elimination, rebuild, revitalize, cleanse the blood and lungs, strengthen and stabilize the nervous system. In conjunction with asana and pranayama, Yoga hygiene, nutrition, and periodic fasting are utilized in the thorough cleansing program. (With respect to the "health" aspect of pranayama it should be pointed out here that although breath suspension would appear to decrease the amount of oxygen absorbed, the respiratory system is so conditioned during pranayama that, following its practice, larger amounts of oxygen are absorbed for a longer period of time than would ordinarily be the case. Further, Yogis maintain that respiration that is regulated and slowed promotes longevity. They point to the fact that those animals which breathe the slowest are the longest-lived.)

In the process of respiration two principal *currents* or *impulses* (*vayus*) are generated that are of primary importance in Hatha Yoga. They are known respectively as the *prana vayu* and *apana vayu* and operate in the organism in a way that may be considered as afferent and efferent. The prana vayu is a current or impulse that collects in the area of the heart and continually *ascends,* circulating in the upper regions of the body, including the brain. The apana vayu collects in the area of the solar plexus from where it continually *decends* and circulates in the lower regions, including the anus. The prana vayu is the *conserving* current; conservation is cool and positive in nature; it is designated symbolically as the lunar (moon) principle and to it is applied the Sanskrit syllable "ha." The apana vayu is the *consuming* current; consumption is equated with heat; it is designated as the solar (sun) principle and to it is applied the Sanskrit syllable "tha."

The prana and apana vayus, then, manifest a positive-negative situation: they continually pull against one another and are in conflict. According to the tenets of Hatha Yoga the continual restlessness that is experienced in the organism (body and mind) is due to this conflict or discord between the prana and apana vayus. The principal objective of Hatha Yoga, therefore, becomes the uniting, the concordance or harmonization of the two currents. The procedure to achieve this objective is as follows: asana, pranayama, and attendant practices, (hygiene, diet, etc.) are undertaken to properly cleanse and strengthen the subtle and physical systems. When this has been accomplished certain of the techniques of pranayama (accompanied by *mudras*) will effect a *reversal* of the unchecked tendencies of the prana and apana: the prana is made to move *downward* (instead of upward) and the apana is made to move *upward* in such a way that they meet and join with each other. This union is "sealed" or "locked" through the application of *bandhas*.

In the network of nadis, three are considered as primary: *ida, pingala,* and *sushumna.* Fig. M depicts their locations. Sushumna extends from the Muladhara to the Ajna; it passes through the center of the chakras. In the sushumna there are two additional nadis enclosed within one another and it is the "tube" within the finest of these that is the actual conduit for the kundalini. Ida and pingala receive their supply of prana through the process of respiration and are connected to the left and right nostrils respectively. They intertwine the sushumna in a serpentine pattern and both extend from the Muladhara to the Ajna (meeting sushumna at both of these chakras). Prana, therefore, is continually circulating through the ida and pingala. (The word "prana" is used to designate both the basic life-force element—a major source of which is respiration—*and* the ascending vayu, the prana vayu. The reader must note the distinction.)

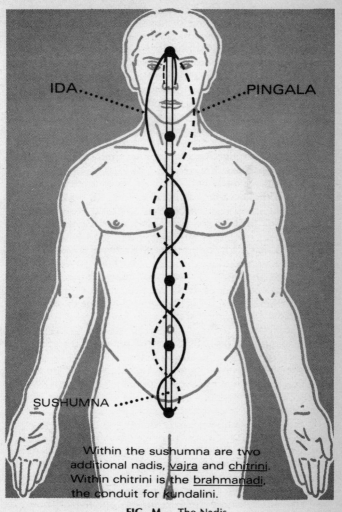

IDA .... PINGALA

SUSHUMNA ....

Within the sushumna are two
additional nadis, vajra and chitrini.
Within chitrini is the brahmanadi,
the conduit for kundalini.

FIG. M — The Nadis

When the prana vayu and the apana vayu are made to meet, and this union is "sealed," they are directed by the consciousness to the Muladhara center at the base of the spine that is the entrance to the sushumna nadi (the spinal canal). In the ordinary man the sushumna nadi is closed and remains so throughout his lifetime. *The Hatha Yoga student must open the sushumna;* this is accomplished by gently "pushing" the prana into it at its base. Through the continued application of cleansing, asana, mudra, pranayama, and concentration-meditation the student is eventually able to totally withdraw the prana from ida and pingala and direct it into the sushumna. In other words, ida and pingala, the two principal circuits of prana are devitalized; their prana is withdrawn and *made to enter the central spinal canal.* Once this is accomplished respiration is automatically suspended and all flow of thoughts (*vrittis*) is halted; the ripples are stilled, the body, breath, and mind rest. Throughout the time the student is practicing to unite the prana and apana vayus he increases his concentration capabilities. But when the vayus are made to unite at the Muladhara chakra and the prana enters the central spinal canal (sushumna), concentration-meditation can be undertaken to great advantage. In the context of *this* presentation of Hatha Yoga the above two processes (unification of the vayus and prana entrance into the sushumna) are the ultimate objectives.

The length of time that the breath (prana) can be made to remain in the sushumna will increase as the student gains proficiency in the techniques that are involved. In this regard, the continual cleansing of the nadis, through regular practice, cannot be overemphasized.

The reader can now understand that asana, pranayama, and the attendant practices that comprise the system of Hatha Yoga were developed to achieve its major objectives: uniting the vayus and directing the prana into the central spinal canal. *The health benefits that are experienced in the course of these practices are actually by-products!* He can also understand how the name of this system of Yoga was derived: the entrance of the prana into the sushumna is accomplished through the uniting (Yoga) of the two vayus—solar and lunar, positive and negative—that are known respectively through imposition of the Sanskrit syllables "ha" and "tha." Thus, unification (Yoga) of "ha" and "tha" becomes HA/THA YOGA.

At that stage where prana can be made to enter and remain for a period of time in the sushumna, Hatha Yoga functions in conjunction with Raja Yoga through the pursuit of those concentration-meditation practices that comprise the sixth, seventh, and eighth limbs of the Patanjali structure. But also at this point the Laya practices can be undertaken—in lieu of Raja—to awaken the kundalini shakti and raise it through the chakras (chapter 5). However, as we have previously stated, Laya is comprised of a series of extremely advanced practices and presupposes complete control of various systems of the physical and subtle bodies. Since the achievement of such control by the student will first require his expenditure of considerable time and effort in perfecting the techniques presented in the following pages, it is imprudent to detail the Laya practices in this book. Nonetheless, to prepare the chakras for the awakening of kundalini, their yantras are included among the geometric forms that are to be visualized by the student during his Hatha practice.

Is it necessary to practice Hatha to achieve the objectives of Yoga in general? We have stated that, due to the manner in which the ordinary mind functions, the student often encounters difficulty in sustaining not only his awareness of the conspiracy but his incentive to practice with the seriousness and regularity that are necessary. However, because of its profound effects on his organism, the student *enjoys and anticipates Hatha practice;* that is, in desiring to maintain that exhilarating physiological experience which results from Hatha, his organism all but *compels* him to apply its techniques regularly. Each practice session, by totally capturing his attention for a certain period of time, automatically reinforces for him many of the Yogic principles that have been outlined in these pages. In this process Yoga becomes more and more a part of his everyday life. Hatha, therefore, not only offers a most expeditious entrance into Yoga on a continuing basis and is extremely supportive of all other Yogas, but, in itself, is able to escort the student far along the path to the ultimate Yoga objectives. Consequently, Hatha practice is highly recommended by the author.

Chapter 2

Hatha Yoga:
The Practice

In this chapter we offer a comprehensive course in Hatha Yoga. The reader who undertakes the program seriously can expect to:

Experience those health benefits heretofore described;

Quiet and steady the ordinary mind;

Render the consciousness fit for productive concentration-meditation;

Prepare the physical and subtle bodies for the esoteric objectives of Hatha Yoga.

The following instructions for practice should be very carefully observed:

- The time of the day selected for practice is left to the student's discretion. Ideally, upon arising, a few minutes will be spent in gently loosening the body with several of the mild stretching movements, followed by a brief period of pranayama and concentration or meditation. The full practice will be undertaken at any convenient time later in the day when the body has become more flexible. Practicing at approximately the same hour each day is highly recommended; practice directly prior to retiring is not advised.

- Practice is ideal with the stomach empty; at least ninety minutes should elapse after meals before practice is begun.

- Choose a place of privacy where disturbances are minimal. Fresh air, even in cold weather, is essential. A flat surface is necessary.

- Practice clothing should permit complete freedom of movement. There should be nothing restricting on the body; glasses, jewelry, and watch should be removed.

- A mat is required. The color and design should be quiet and relaxing. This should be used *only* for Yoga practice.

- The beginning student must be content to assume only the most elementary positions of the asanas and *very gradually* progress into the intermediate and advanced positions. The period of time that may be required to "progress" is of no consequence. When the body is ready it will move into the next stage; if the student strains in any way to prematurely "progress" he will actually retard genuine progress.

- If there is any concern as to the physical effects of the practice on one who has a history of illness, a physician should be consulted prior to beginning.

The beginning student should spend some weeks in getting the "feel" of the asanas *without* applying breath retention or visualization. He must attempt to develop slow-motion rhythm, gracefulness, and poise in all movements.

Regardless of the degree of proficiency that is attained it is *always* advisable to "warm up" during any given practice session by performing the asanas at least once in an elementary position without breath retention.

Once the execution of the techniques has been correctly learned it is advisable to *lower* the eyelids so that just a slit of light remains. By so doing we avoid visual distractions but do not simulate sleep. The photographs below depict the models performing the asanas with the eyes open (for the beginning student who is in the process of carefully learning the movements) and the eyelids lowered (for the more advanced student).

The directions for respiration in the asanas that follow are in italics. These must be carefully studied and observed. All directions should be read at each practice session until there is not the slightest doubt as to the correct execution of the techniques. Precision, in Yoga, is essential. However, regardless of the directions, the student must never maintain the extreme position or retain the breath for one second longer than is comfortable. Once there is absolutely no strain in retaining for the indicated number of seconds, the student may *very gradually add seconds* to this retention time.

Learn to approximate "seconds" in counting. For longer holding periods, as in the Shoulder and Head Stands, a timepiece should be placed where it may be easily read.

No technique is to be neglected; each is to be practiced exactly as presented in the Groups of the "Practice Guide." The student is in no position to judge what his eventual proficiency may be in any given technique and he should make no attempt to do so. He must simply perform each technique to the best of his ability during each practice session. The *practice*, not concern with the attainment of an ultimate position, is what is called for.

The consciousness is to be occupied in one of two ways during the practice: (1) It is directed to that area where the maximum stretch, pull, weight, etc., is experienced. This directing of the consciousness and "feeling" of the emphasized area, to the exclusion of all other thoughts and sensations, effectively stabilizes and calms the ordinary mind and increases the physical benefits of the practice. (2) It "visualizes" the yantras (simplified forms of the chakras) and other geometric forms. This is a concentration practice that prepares the subtle body for activation of the kundalini and renders the consciousness fit for meditation. The student should not undertake the visualization practice until he is accomplished in directing his consciousness to the various areas of the organism as described in (1).

The application of (1) maintains the "physical" dimension of the Hatha practice. The application of (2) —in conjunction with breath suspension—transforms the physical practice into that which is "spiritual." The procedure for both techniques is given in the directions that follow. The photographs clearly indicate that area of the organism which is being emphasized and is, therefore, to be "felt," and that geometric form which is to be visualized. The elementary student is to follow the instructions for directing his consciousness to the indicated area of the body regardless of his degree of attainment. For example, if, in a particular asana, he is instructed to direct his consciousness to the base of the spine and to "feel" that area, he must follow this instruction even though, as a beginning student, his performance of the asana does not yet enable him to experience the full physical emphasis at that point.

It is perfectly acceptable if, in a given practice session, the accomplished student applies (1) in his first execution of an asana or mudra, and then applies (2) in the repetitions of that asana or mudra.

Those readers who are interested in the very specific physical and therapeutic objectives of the asanas should consult my book *Introduction to Yoga*.

HALF-LOTUS (Accomplished Posture; Siddhasana)

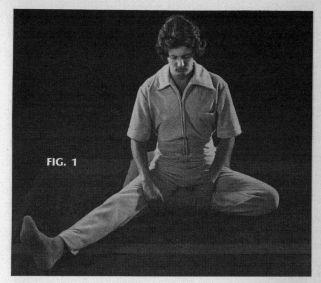

FIG. 1

FIG. 1 — The use of a pillow that provides approximately six inches of sitting height is desirable although not essential. Sit with the legs extended. The hands place the left foot so that the heel is against the perineum and the sole against the right thigh.

PHYSICAL EFFECTS OF LOTUS POSTURES: promotes flexibility of the knees, ankles and feet; develops the ability to remain firmly and quietly seated for periods of meditation.

Each time the Half-Lotus is assumed the student should direct his consciousness through his body to check the following:

Slight pressure against perineum with left heel (this pressure to be maintained).

Slight pressure against pubic bone with right heel (this pressure to be maintained).

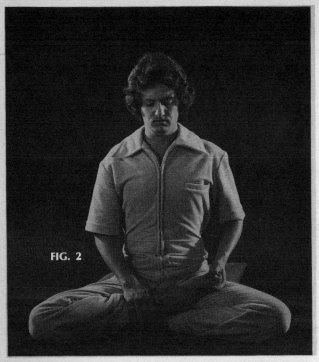

FIG. 2 — Place the right heel against the pubic bone.

The right foot rests on the left thigh as illustrated. Note that the sole is turned upward as far as possible.

The male student must adjust the genitals as necessary to achieve this position without discomfort.

Slight pressure in the touching of the thumbs and index fingers (this pressure to be maintained).

Trunk and head erect but relaxed; eyelids lowered.

The beginning student can practice by placing first the right foot on top of the left thigh as instructed above, and then, when this becomes uncomfortable, exchanging the position of the legs. However, he should concentrate on perfecting the traditional position, which is that of the right foot on top.

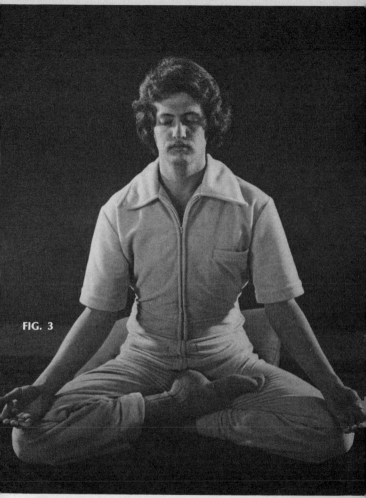

FIG. 3

FIG. 3 — The trunk and head are erect but relaxed. The eyelids are lowered, not closed. The hands rests on the knees with the thumbs touching the index fingers, palms turned upward. There is a slight pressure in the touching of the thumb and index finger and this pressure is maintained as long as the student is seated in the posture.

LOTUS (Padmasana)

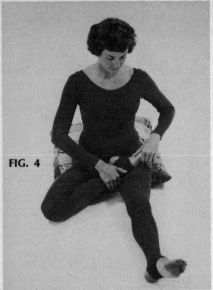

FIG. 4 — Use of the pillow is desirable.

Sit with the legs extended. The hands place the right foot on the left thigh so that the right heel presses gently into the groin.

The following should be checked:

Slight pressure against the groin with both heels (this pressure to be maintained).

Correct hand position with slight pressure in the contact (to be maintained).

Trunk and head erect but relaxed; eyelids lowered (not closed). Again, the beginning student, to aid in making the legs supple, may reverse the position of the feet. However, the position instructed above is the one to be perfected.

Preliminary practice for the Lotus: One foot is placed on the opposite thigh while slight pressure is exerted by the forearm resting on the knee. Remain in this position for two to three minutes. Then practice with the other leg. The knees will gradually lower.

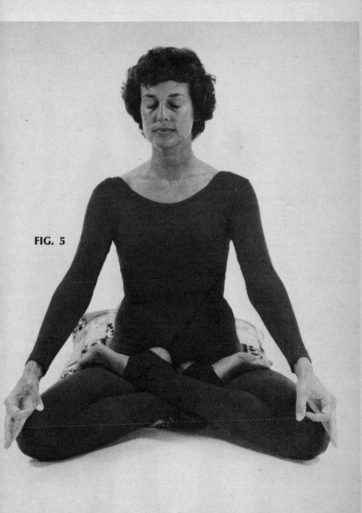

FIG. 5

FIG. 5 — The left foot is placed on the right thigh so that the left heel presses gently into the groin.
The heels are brought close together, the feet turned upward.

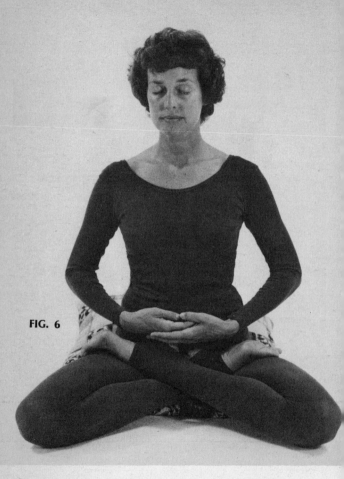

FIG. 6

FIG. 6 — The hands may be placed in three possible positions: as in the Half-Lotus; as above in Fig. 5; as illustrated here, where the left hand rests upon the heels and the right hand rests firmly in the left.

SIMPLE POSTURE (Sukhasana)

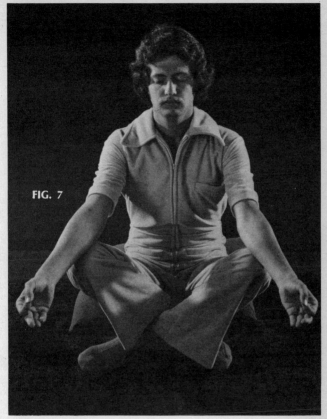

FIG. 7

FIG. 7; FIG. 8 — The pillow can be used.
Cross the ankles (either may be on top) and draw the
legs in as far as possible.
Hands are placed as in the Half-Lotus.
Trunk and head are erect but relaxed.
Eyelids are lowered.

This position is for the student who is practicing to
accomplish the preceding two positions but, as yet,
finds them too difficult for comfortable practice.

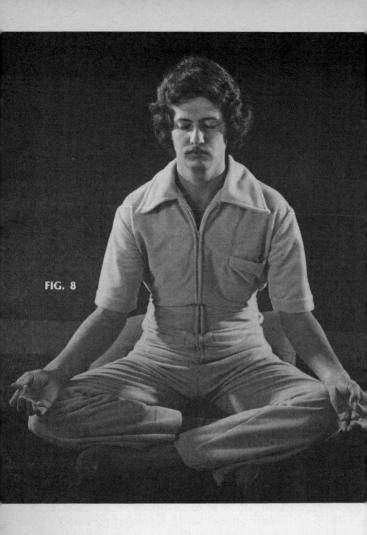

FIG. 8

PHYSICAL EFFECTS: increases lung capacity and oxygenation; revitalizes; promotes alertness and clarity of mind.

COMPLETE BREATH

Most of the asanas that follow are performed in conjunction with a form of breath control that is known as the "Complete Breath." Accordingly, we must learn the technique at this point. Certain physical movements, aside from the movements of the asana itself, must be coordinated with inhalation, retention, and exhalation. It is these movements that make this form of breathing deep and full, that is, *complete*.

Sit in a cross-legged posture. Breathe normally.

Practice a few moments to gain control of the abdominal muscles.

First expand the abdomen by pushing down with the diaphragm and use the abdominal muscles to slowly extend the abdomen (Fig. 9).

Then use these muscles to slowly contract the abdomen (Fig. 10).

Continue to expand and contract until you have control of these muscles.

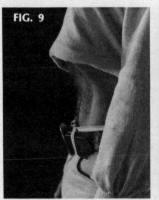 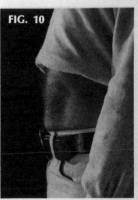

FIG. 9 — Exhale slowly and deeply. Contract the abdomen to aid in completely expelling the air from the lungs.

FIG. 10 — Begin a slow, deep, quiet inhalation through the nose (all breathing is done through the nose in this course). This inhalation is taken so quietly that you can scarcely feel the air entering your nostrils. During this inhalation the abdomen is slowly expanded.

In the beginning stages of your Yoga practice, continue to perform this Complete Breath at each practice session until it is second nature and the physical movements flow easily into one another while respiration continues independently of them. When perfected, the inhalations and exhalations should require approximately seven seconds each and the retention will be dependent upon the length of time that the extreme position of the asana is held.

Whenever, in the following asanas, you are directed to "inhale," "retain," "exhale," it is the movements of this Complete Breath that are indicated.

Mudras—Bandhas

Mudras are techniques that profoundly influence the pranic currents (vayus). The contact of the index fingers and thumbs in the Lotus postures is a mudra. There are nine mudras among the techniques instructed in the following pages; the student should note that these are mudras and not confuse them with the asanas. The nine are: Abdominal Lift, Alternate Leg Pull, Head Stand, Raised Lotus, Locked Lotus, Yoga Mudra, and the three bandhas. When perfected these are applied for the purposes of uniting the prana and apana vayus and directing them into the sushumna.

Bandhas are mudras that are applied for the specific purpose of *binding* or *sealing* the unification of the prana and apana. The three bandhas to be learned at this point are: Chin-Lock, Abdominal Contraction, and Anal Contraction.

FIG. 11 — Without disrupting the inhalation, which continues to flow quietly and smoothly, slowly expand the chest. As the chest is expanded the abdomen is to be slightly contracted. Complete the inhalation as the chest is fully expanded.

Retain the air. Begin with a five-second retention and gradually increase the duration to twenty seconds.

Exhale slowly, quietly, deeply. No sound is made in the nostrils and no special movements are necessary for the exhalation other than relaxing the chest and abdomen. When the exhalation is almost complete, contract the abdomen to aid in expelling all air from the lungs.

Repeat without pause.

Concentration will be wholly on perfecting the technique.

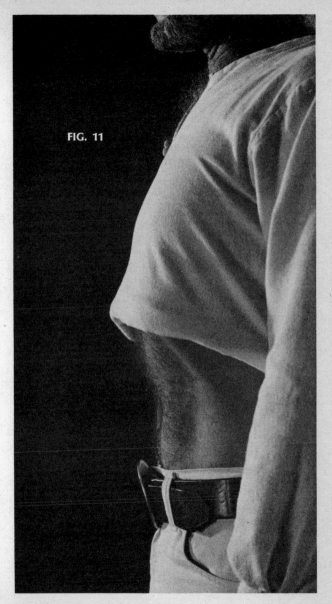

FIG. 11

CHIN-LOCK

FIG. 12 — Close the throat (glottis) by contracting the vocal chords. This is easy to do. Simply make the constricting movement in the throat that will prevent air from entering or leaving.

Then, keeping the throat closed, and with the spine erect, press the chin tightly against the uppermost area of the chest.

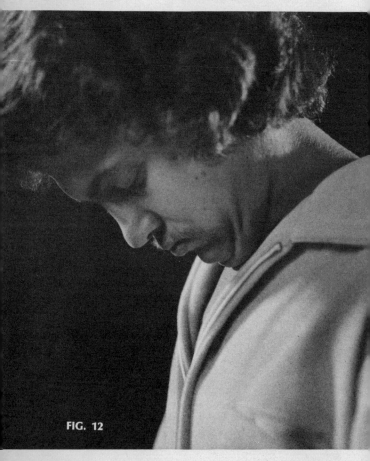

FIG. 12

ABDOMINAL CONTRACTION

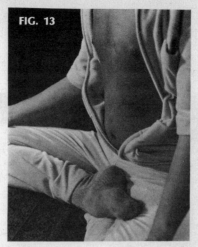

FIG. 13 — The abdomen is in a normal, relaxed position.

FIG. 14 — The abdominal muscles have contracted to draw and hold the abdomen inward as far as possible.

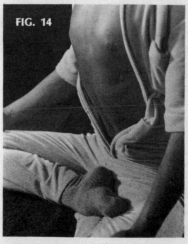

ANAL CONTRACTION

The rectum is held closed by a forcible contraction of the anal sphincters.

SIMULTANEOUS APPLICATION OF THE BANDHAS

FIG. 15 — Sit in Siddhasana (Half-Lotus), or, if necessary, in the Simple posture. Lower the eyelids. Make certain that the heels are exerting pressure in the proper areas.

Press the tongue firmly against the root of the two front center teeth and hold it there.

Suspend respiration without any special inhalation or exhalation. That is, simply stop breathing.

Apply and hold the Chin-Lock.

Apply and hold the Abdominal Contraction.

Apply and hold the Anal Contraction.

Prana is now locked within the body. Maintain the position long enough to get the "feel" of the bandhas.

Raise the head and resume respiration.

Relax the tongue; relax the abdomen; relax the anal sphincters.

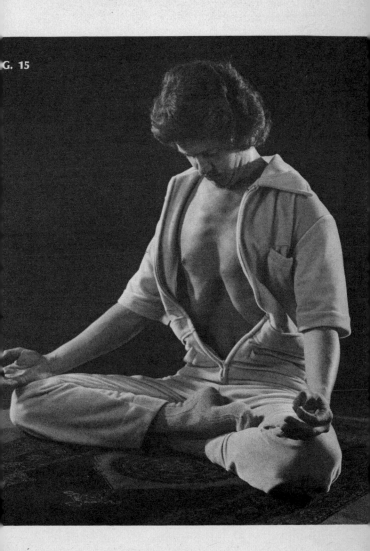

1. COMPLETE BREATH STANDING

(Beginning with this asana all breathing directions appear in italics.)

This technique combines the Complete Breath with the body movements indicated below and the simultaneous visualization of a continual passive-active cycle.

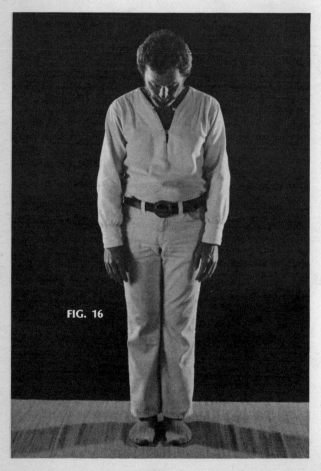

FIG. 16

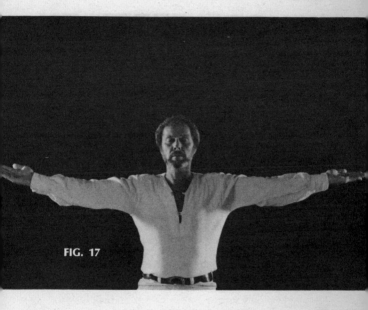

FIG. 17

FIG. 16 — *Exhale deeply* and stand as indicated. This stance represents an attitude of depletion wherein a minimum of life-force is present. Feel and visualize this passive state.

FIG. 17 — The eyes are partially closed and can remain this way throughout the movements. *Begin a very deep, very slow inhalation.* As you inhale expand your abdomen in the manner already learned.

Begin to raise the arms, slowly, palms up. As life-force (prana) enters the lungs the organism is activated, it stirs. Feel and visualize this birth of activity.

FIG. 18 — *Continue the deep, slow inhalation* and the slow raising of the arms. (If the inhalation is not performed very slowly and very deeply it will be completed before you can perform the necessary physical movements.) Now the chest expands and as more air enters the lungs and more life-force fills the body you become increasingly "alive."

As the palms meet overhead the *inhalation is completed.* The lungs are full, the chest expanded, the abdomen slightly contracted. *Retain the air* for a count of five. Feel and visualize the body being permeated with life-force and totally alive.

Begin a very slow exhalation. The movements are now reversed. The arms are slowly lowered, palms facing down. As the exhalation continues, the life-force is depleted and the body becomes increasingly limp. Feel and visualize this progression. *When the exhalation is completed* the arms rest once again at the sides and the organism should be felt and visualized in a passive state. There is no breathing for several seconds. Then the process is repeated.

Perform five times.

With the aid of the breathing and physical movements we practice to feel and visualize a continuous, smooth progression from the static to the dynamic and back to the static state. By "experiencing" this cycle in an abbreviated and repetitious fashion we gain a perspective of the passive-active-passive-active pattern that is extremely meaningful in the overall objective of our work.

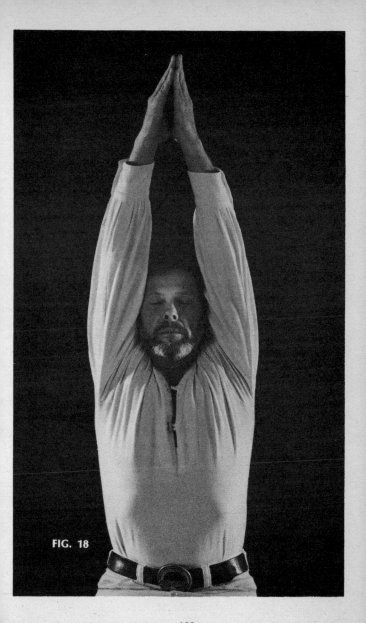

FIG. 18

2. CHEST EXPANSION
(Ardha Chakrasana)

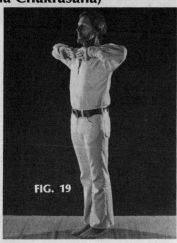

FIG. 19

FIG. 19; FIG. 20 — Stand with your heels together, arms at sides. Your eyes are partially closed and remain this way throughout the movements. *Begin a slow, deep inhalation.* In very slow, graceful motion bring your hands up so that they touch your chest.

Slowly stretch your arms straight outward as far as possible.

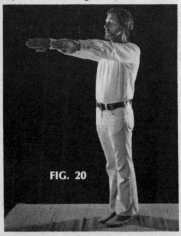

FIG. 20

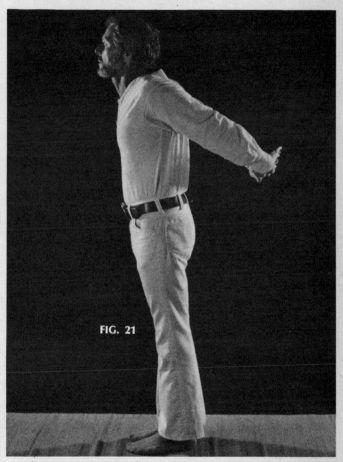

FIG. 21

FIG. 21 — *Continue the slow, deep inhalation.* Slowly bring the arms back. Hold them high, on a level with your shoulders and interlace the fingers. *Complete the inhalation at this point.*

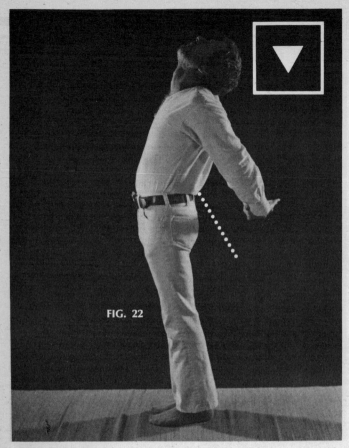

FIG. 22 — *Retain the air.* Very cautiously bend as far backward as possible. The arms are held high. Hold the position approximately ten seconds. Direct the consciousness to the base of the spine. *Feel* this area. Practice visualizing the illustrated figure (the Muladhara chakra).

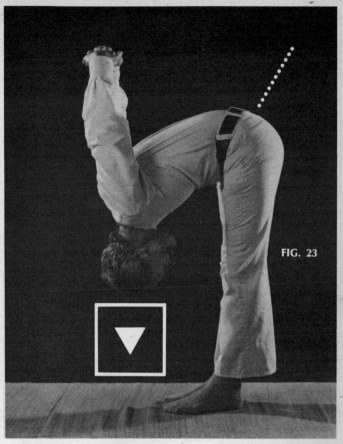

FIG. 23

FIG. 23 — *Retaining the air,* slowly straighten upright. *Begin a slow exhalation.* Very slowly bend as far forward as possible, continuing the exhalation. In your extreme forward position *the exhalation is completed and thereafter the breathing is normal.* Note the position of the arms and that the neck is completely relaxed. Hold this position motionless for approximately twenty seconds during which you feel and visualize as in Fig. 22.

Straighten up slowly and relax.

Perform twice.

3. RISHI'S POSTURE (Rishiasana)

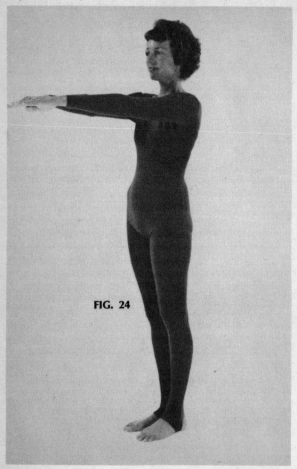

FIG. 24

FIG. 24 — Your eyes remain partially open throughout the movements. Stand with your heels slightly apart and arms at sides. *Begin a slow, deep inhalation.* Slowly raise your arms so that the hands meet in front as illustrated. *Complete the inhalation at this point.*

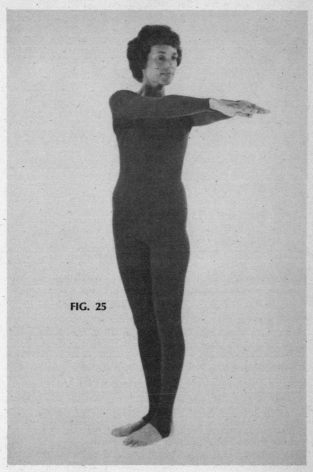

FIG. 25

FIG. 25 — *Retain the air*. Slowly turn your head, trunk, and arms ninety degrees to the left. Arms move at shoulder level and eyes remain fixed on the hands.

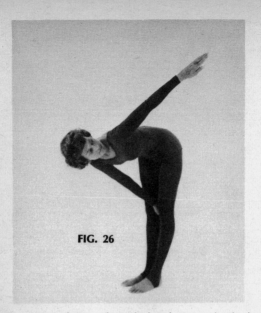

FIG. 26

FIG. 26 — *Retain the air*. The right hand moves slowly down the *inside* of the right leg. The left arm moves behind you with the head also turning to the left. Eyes follow the left hand. Knees remain straight.

FIG. 27 — *Retain the air*. The left arm has moved to the overhead position while the right hand has moved to the bottom of the right leg and holds the right heel. The head has turned as far to the left as possible. Hold this position motionless for ten seconds. During the hold, direct the consciousness to the base of the spine. *Feel* this area. Practice visualizing a cross that has been approximated by the position of the arms, trunk, and head.

Begin the exhalation. Slowly straighten to the upright position, lowering the left arm to the side and raising the right arm to the side. *Complete the exhalation* as the upright position is reached. *Without pause* begin the next inhalation and once again raise the arms. Complete the inhalation, turn slowly to the *right,* and perform the identical movements (with breath retention and visualization of the cross), exchanging the words "right" and "left" in the above directions.

Perform the left-right movements three times.

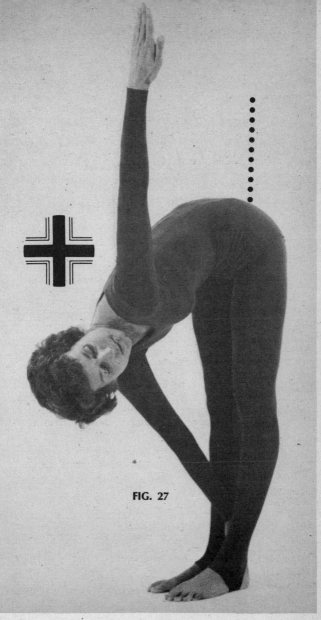

FIG. 27

4. TRIANGLE (Trikonasana)

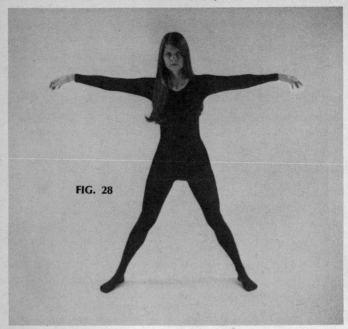

FIG. 28

FIG. 28 — Remember the partial opening of the eyes. Assume a wide stance, arms at sides. *Begin the inhalation* and slowly raise the arms, palms down, to the position illustrated. *Complete the inhalation at this point.*

PHYSICAL EFFECTS: firms the sides and thighs; removes excess weight and inches from the waist.

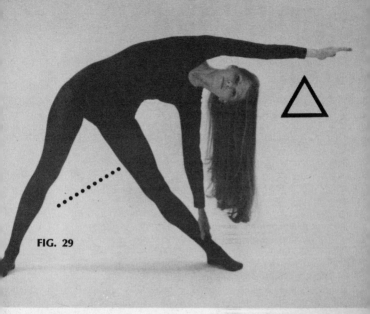

FIG. 29 — *Retain the air*. Slowly bend to the *left* and take a firm hold on your ankle. Neck is relaxed, head is down.

Retain the air. Pull on the ankle and lower the trunk as far as possible. The right arm is above your head and parallel with the floor. Hold for approximately fifteen seconds. During the hold *feel* the stretching throughout the right side and in the upper thighs. The position of the legs makes a triangular figure. Practice visualizing a triangle.

Begin the exhalation and slowly straighten to the upright position. The legs remain apart. Lower your arms to the sides and *complete the exhalation at this point. Without pause* begin the next inhalation and once again raise the arms. Complete the inhalation, bend to the *right*, and perform the identical movements on the right side (with breath retention and visualization of the triangle).

Perform the left-right movements three times.

Slowly straighten to the upright position. Gracefully lower your arms to the sides and draw the legs together. Relax.

5. BALANCE POSTURE (Natarajasana)

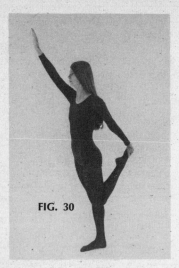

FIG. 30

FIG. 30 — The eyes remain partially open throughout. In a standing position with heels together, *begin the inhalation.* Slowly and gracefully raise your right arm.

Continuing the inhalation, shift your weight onto the right leg. Bend your left knee and raise your left leg so that the left hand can hold the left foot as illustrated. *Complete the inhalation at this point.*

FIG. 31 — *Retain the air.* Pull your left foot upward; move your right arm to the overhead position; drop your head back. Hold with as little motion as possible for ten seconds. During the hold *feel* the stretching in the abdominal area and the middle of the spine.

Practice visualizing the elements of the Manipura chakra as illustrated.

Begin the exhalation. Release the foot and return it slowly to the floor; simultaneously lower the right arm to the side. *Complete the exhalation at this point.*

Without pause begin the next inhalation. Execute the identical movements with *left* arm and *right* foot raised.

Perform twice, alternating sides.

144

PHYSICAL EFFECTS: develops poise and equilibrium.

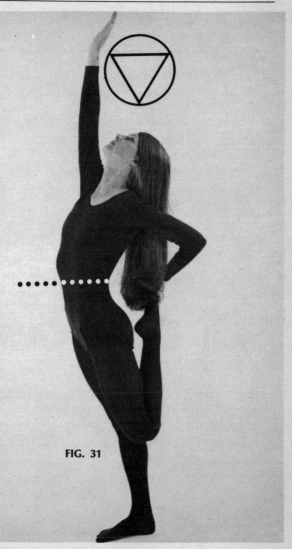

FIG. 31

6. ABDOMINAL LIFT (Uddiyana)

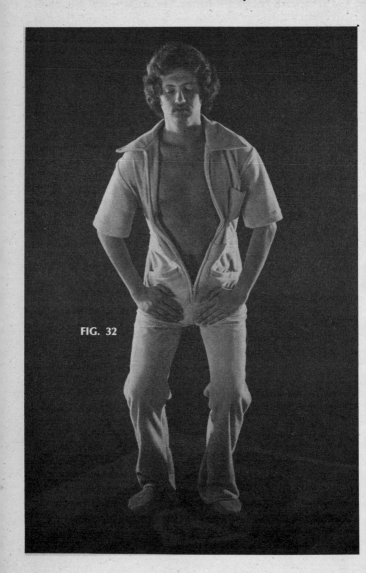

FIG. 32

PHYSICAL EFFECTS: tones the abdominal muscles; removes excess abdominal weight; stimulates the organs of the viscera.

FIG. 32 — Study the illustration carefully, because the correct position in this technique is extremely important. The feet are apart, knees bent slightly outward, hands pressed firmly against the upper thighs, fingers (including thumbs) together and turned inward. The trunk is lowered several inches but remains straight; do not bend forward.

FIG. 33; FIG. 34 — Fig. 33 and Fig. 34 depict the completed Abdominal Lift. Note that the abdomen is not simply contracted, but *lifted*. This lift requires gaining control of the abdominal muscles and the emptying of the lungs through a deep and complete exhalation prior to the lift. You cannot raise the abdomen into the proper position unless the lungs are first emptied and remain empty for the duration of the lift.

Assume the stance, as illustrated. *Exhale deeply and retain the air out of your lungs.* This creates the necessary vacuum. Close your throat so that no air can pass through it. Now imagine that you are going to take a deep breath from the pit of your stomach: use your abdominal muscles as you would your lungs, so that the abdomen is "sucked" inward and upward (of course, no air is permitted to enter; this is a deep "breath" with the abdominal muscles only).

Hold the lift (or, in the beginning stages, a simple contraction will suffice) for a second or two and then quickly and forcefully "snap" the abdomen out. Begin with five lifts per exhalation and work up to twenty-five or more lifts per exhalation. Each exhalation, together with its lifts, constitutes one round. When you have completed each round, *inhale deeply,* straighten upright slowly, and relax for a few seconds, breathing normally.

Your eyes remain partially open during the movements. The point of physical concentration is, of course, the abdomen. Practice visualizing, as in the Balance posture, the Manipura chakra (navel center).

Perform five rounds of the lifts.

When relaxing briefly between rounds continue the visualization of the Manipura chakra.

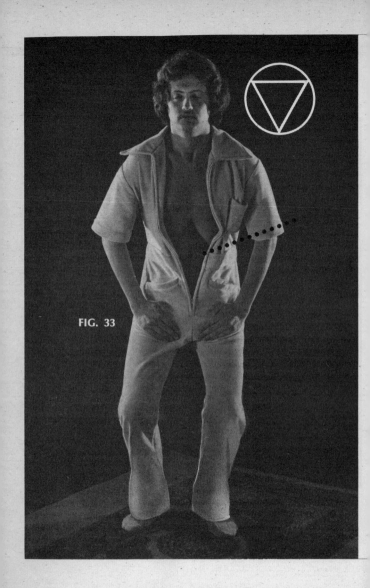

FIG. 33

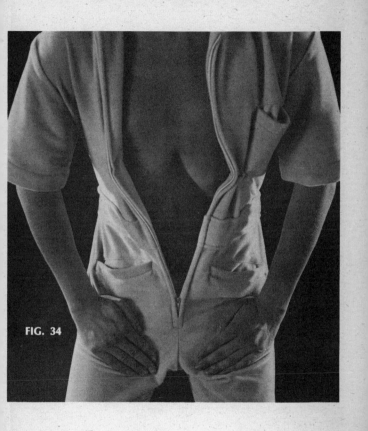

FIG. 34

7. TWIST (Ardha Matsyendrasana)

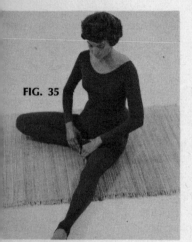

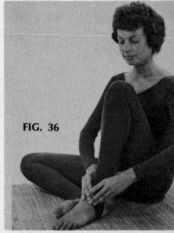

FIG. 35

FIG. 36

FIG. 35 — In a seated position, lower your eyelids to the usual position and extend your legs straight outward.
Take hold of your right foot and bring the heel as far in as possible; the sole rests flat against your upper left thigh.

FIG. 36 — Bring your left leg in so that you can take a firm hold of your left ankle with both hands.

PHYSICAL EFFECTS: provides immediate relief of stiffness in the spine; tones the muscles of the back; promotes flexibility.

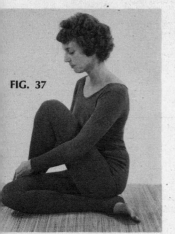
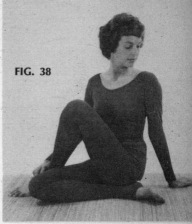

FIG. 37 — Study the photograph. You now swing your left foot over your right knee and place it firmly on the floor adjacent to your right thigh.

FIG. 38 — Remove the left hand from the ankle and place it firmly on the floor behind you for support.

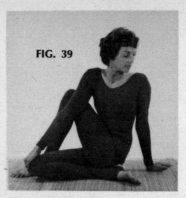

FIG. 39

FIG. 39 — Remove your right hand from your ankle and slowly bring it *over* your left leg.

Take a firm hold on your right knee with your right hand. (Some adjustments of the leg and trunk may be necessary to accomplish this position.)

FIG. 40 — *Inhale and retain.* In this twisted position a deep inhalation will be difficult but can be accomplished with some practice. Very slowly turn your trunk and head as far to your *left* as possible. Simultaneously move your left hand from the floor to hold the right side of your waist. Study the photograph. Note that the head is turned far to the left, as though you would rest your chin on your shoulder. At first this position will feel tight, cramped, uncomfortable, but the body adjusts to it after just a few practice sessions. Hold without motion for ten seconds (you are also retaining the air). During the hold direct the consciousness along the spine and *feel* the corkscrewlike shape in which it has been placed. For visualization, construct a spiral figure in an ascending direction.

Place your left palm back down on the floor and slowly turn your trunk forward so that you have returned to the position of Fig. 38. *Exhale deeply.* Relax a few seconds. Inhale again and repeat the twisting movements.

Return to the frontward position and extend the legs.

Perform the identical movements on the opposite side by exchanging the words "right" and "left" in the above directions.

Perform twice to the left side and twice to the right side.

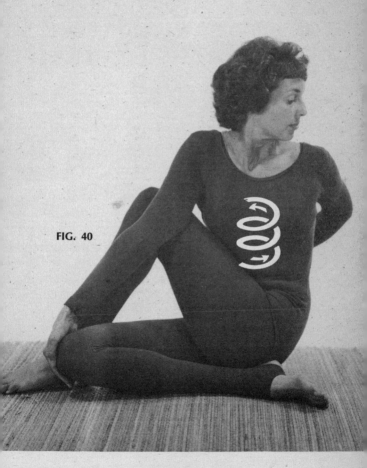

FIG. 40

8. BACKWARD BEND (Supta-Vajrasana)

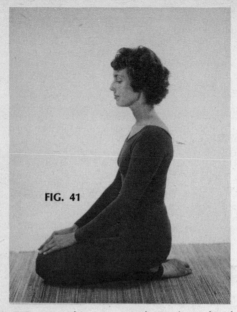

FIG. 41

FIG. 41; FIG. 42 — This asana may be performed with the feet in either position.

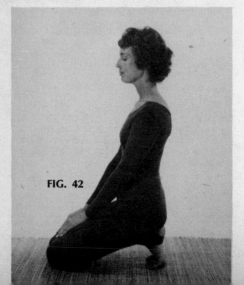

FIG. 42

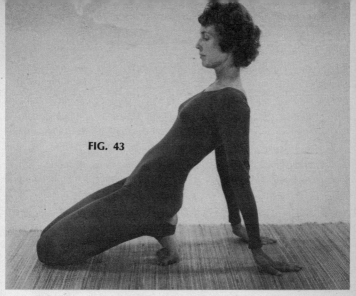

FIG. 43 — In a seated posture, with the eyes in the usual position, place the hands as indicated. Keep the knees together throughout the movements.

FIG. 44 — Slowly and cautiously inch backward with the hands as far as possible. Remain seated on your heels. *Inhale deeply and retain.*

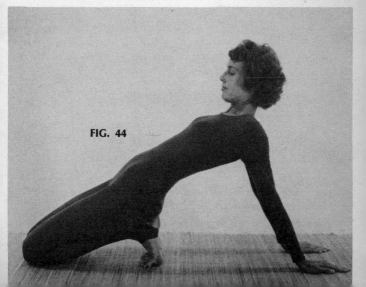

PHYSICAL EFFECTS: strengthens the ankles, feet and toes; promotes flexibility; develops the chest and bust.

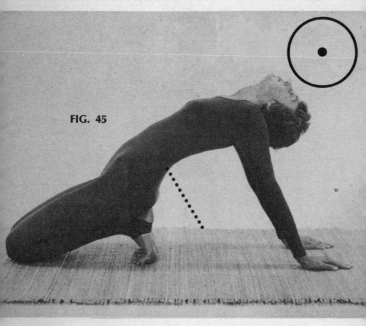

FIG. 45

FIG. 45 — Arch the back and lower the head. Hold motionless for fifteen seconds.

Direct the consciousness to the center of the spine. Practice visualizing a circle with a dot in the center.

Retaining the air, lift the trunk and head. *Exhale deeply*. Relax a few seconds but maintain the posture. Inhale and repeat.

Raise the trunk and head, exhale, and very slowly inch your way forward. Come out of the posture and relax.

Perform twice.

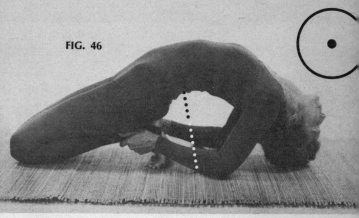

FIG. 46

FIG. 46 — A position for advanced students only which is attained by lowering the elbows (one at a time), forearms, and top of the head to the floor. The breathing and visualization directions are the same.

9. COBRA (Bhujangasana)

PHYSICAL EFFECTS: provides immediate relief of tension throughout the back and spine; promotes deep relaxation and a restful sleep.

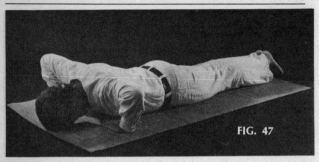

FIG. 47

FIG. 47 — Rest your forehead on the mat and place your hands, with the fingers together, beneath your shoulders. The fingers point directly at the opposite hand. Lower your eyelids and relax all muscles.

Begin a deep inhalation.

FIG. 48 — *Continuing the deep, slow inhalation,* perform these movements in slow motion: arch the neck and raise the head; push against the floor with the hands and raise the trunk. The spine must remain curved and the head must be held back throughout these movements.

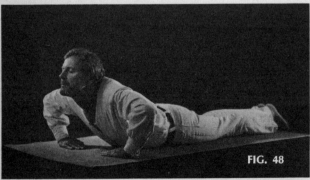

FIG. 48

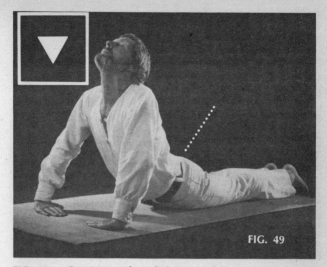

FIG. 49 — *Continuing the inhalation* and keeping the spine curved and the head back, raise the trunk as high as possible without strain. (The ultimate position of the Cobra is depicted in Fig. 49. The elbows are straight, the lower abdomen rests on the floor, and the legs are relaxed.) *Complete the inhalation* as you reach your extreme position. *Retain the air* and hold without motion for twenty seconds.

During the hold *feel* the pressure at the base of the spine.

Practice visualizing the root center, the Muladhara chakra.

Begin the exhalation. (Remember that all exhalations in the asanas are slow, deep and silent; the air is never permitted to rush out uncontrolled.) Now reverse the movements and *slowly* lower the trunk to the floor keeping the spine curved and the head back until the upper chest touches the floor.

Rest your forehead on the mat and *complete the exhalation* at this point.

Relax for approximately one minute with your cheek on the mat and arms at sides. Breathe normally and experience the deep relaxation that the movements of the Cobra impart. Remain aware of this feeling and do not allow the consciousness to wander.

Place your forehead on the mat, begin the inhalation, and repeat.

Perform three times.

10. LOCUST (Salabhasana)

PHYSICAL EFFECTS: develops, strengthens and imparts good muscle tone to the lower abdomen, groin, buttocks and arms.

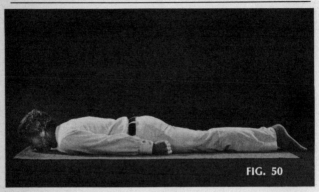

FIG. 50

FIG. 50 — Rest your chin on the mat. Lower the eyelids. Make fists of the hands and place them firmly on the floor, thumbs down, adjacent to your sides.

Inhale and retain.

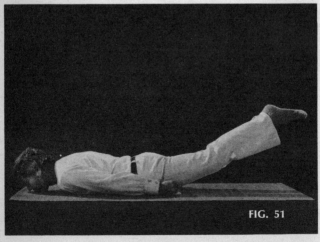

FIG. 51

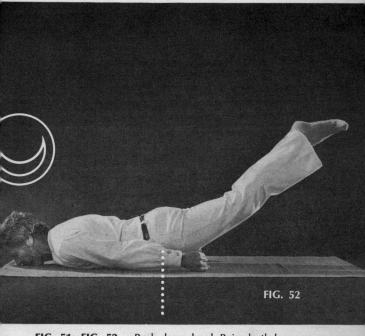

FIG. 52

FIG. 51; FIG. 52 — Push down hard. Raise both legs as high as possible. Fig. 51 depicts a moderate stage and Fig. 53 an advanced one. The chin remains on the mat.

Hold for ten seconds. Direct the consciousness to the groin area.

Practice visualizing the Svadhishthana chakra, the genital center.

Retain the air. Slowly lower the legs to the floor so that you return to the position of Fig. 51. *Exhale with control.* Breathe normally and relax for several seconds. Do not allow the mind to wander.

Inhale and repeat.

Perform three times.

Rest your cheek on the mat and relax.

11. BOW (Dhanurasana)

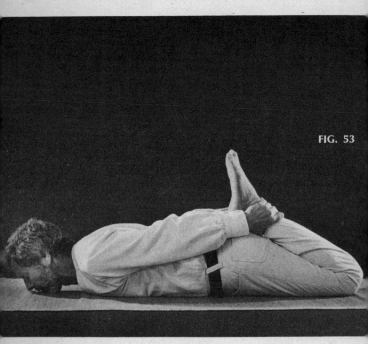

FIG. 53

FIG. 53 — Rest your chin on the mat. Lower the eyelids.
Hold your feet as illustrated. The knees are together.
Inhale and retain.

PHYSICAL EFFECTS: provides intensive strengthening for the back and spine; promotes good posture.

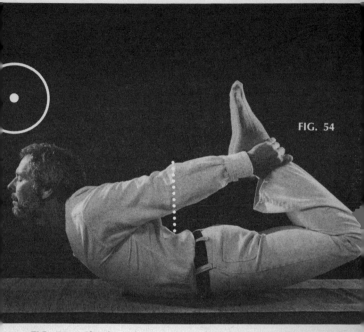

FIG. 54

FIG. 54 — Slowly and cautiously raise the trunk and legs as high as possible. Your head is back and your knees remain together.

Hold motionless for ten seconds. The emphasis should be experienced in the center of the spine. Practice visualizing a circle with a dot in the center.

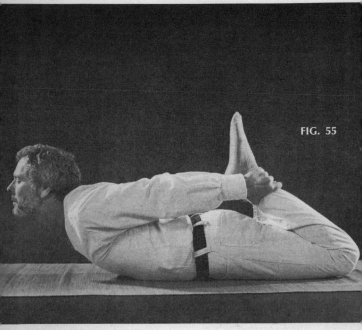

FIG. 55

FIG. 55 — *Retain the air.* First, slowly lower the knees to the floor. Next, slowly lower the trunk and chin to the floor.

Exhale deeply. Breathe normally and relax for several seconds but continue to hold the feet. Do not allow the mind to wander.

Inhale and repeat.

Perform three times.

Following the third exhalation, release the feet and lower them slowly to the floor. Then rest your cheek on the mat and relax.

12. ALTERNATE LEG STRETCH
(Maha Mudra)

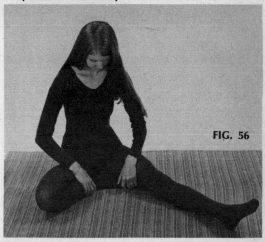

FIG. 56

FIG. 56 — In a seated position lower the eyelids. Extend the left leg and place the right heel so that it exerts pressure on the perineum.

This is the same heel position as in the Half-Lotus. The pressure (without discomfort) is to be maintained throughout these movements.

FIG. 57 — Slowly raise the arms to the position indicated.

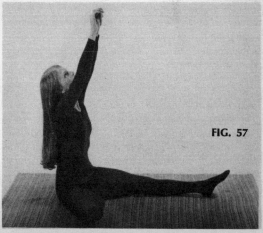

FIG. 57

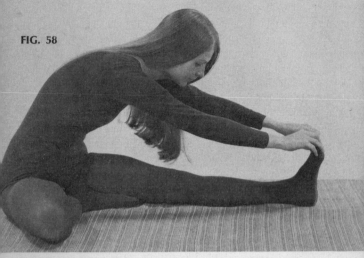

FIG. 58

FIG. 58 — Bend forward slowly and hold the farthest part of the leg that you can reach without strain.

PHYSICAL EFFECTS: firms, strengthens and eliminates tension throughout the legs.

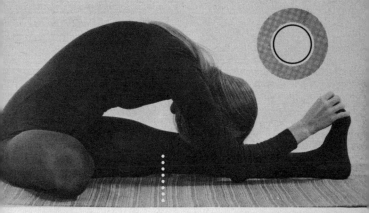

FIG. 59

FIG. 59 — The completed position. Press the forehead against the knee so that pressure is felt between the eyebrows. Your elbows are down, touching the floor if possible.

Inhale and retain. Apply the three bandhas: Chin-Lock, Abdominal and Anal Contractions. Hold for twenty seconds. Check to be sure that pressure is being maintained on the perineum and forehead. Concentrate on the intensive stretching that will occur above the outstretched knee.

Practice visualizing the Ajna chakra, the Mind center.

Begin the slow exhalation. Slowly straighten the trunk to the upright position, simultaneously drawing the hands up the leg.

Complete the exhalation as the trunk becomes upright with the hands resting on the left knee. Relax for several seconds, breathing normally and holding the mind steady.

Repeat.

Perform three times with each leg.

13. SHOULDER STAND (Sarvangasana)

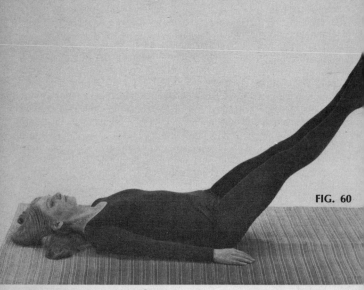

FIG. 60 — In a lying position lower your eyelids, breathe normally. Brace your palms firmly against the floor and raise your legs.

PHYSICAL EFFECTS: improves and aids in regulation of blood pressure and circulation; stimulates the thyroid gland as an aid in weight regulation; relaxes the legs.

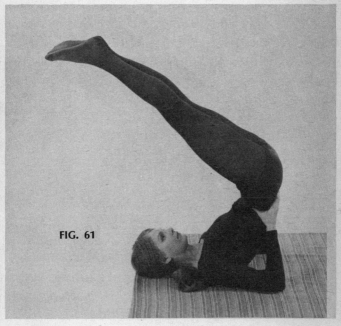

FIG. 61

FIG. 61 — Swing your legs back so that the hips leave the floor. Support the hips with the hands.

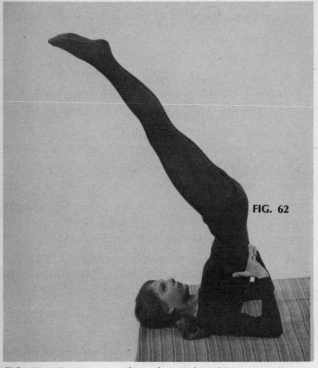

FIG. 62 — Begin to straighten the trunk and legs upward.

FIG. 63 — Continue upward to your extreme position. This is the completed posture. The trunk and legs are straight, forming a right angle with the head. The chin is as close to the chest as possible. The body is relaxed. At first the breathing will be quick and erratic, so practice to normalize it. *There is no breath suspension.*

Begin with a twenty-second hold and work up to five minutes in gradual stages. Maintain the consciousness in the throat and *feel* the increased pressure in this area. Practice visualizing the throat center, the Vishuddha chakra.

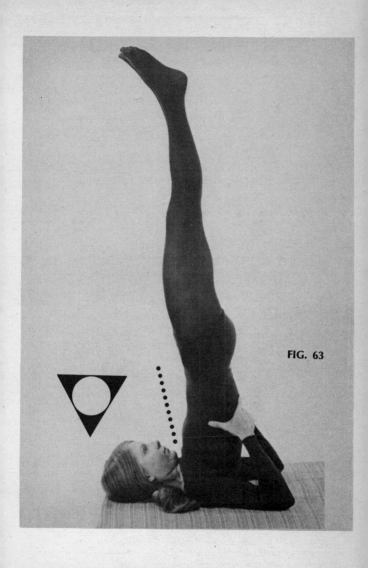

FIG. 63

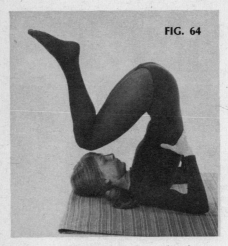

FIG. 64

FIG. 64 — Lower your knees toward your head.

FIG. 65 — Place your palms firmly against the floor. Arch your neck so that your head remains on the floor and roll forward with control.

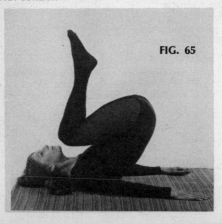

FIG. 65

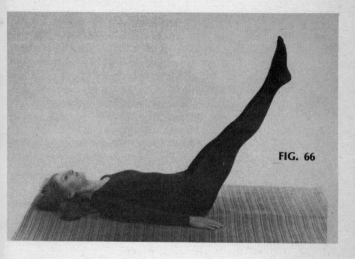

FIG. 66

FIG. 66; FIG. 67 — Extend the legs upward and lower them slowly to the floor. Relax.

The Shoulder Stand is performed once.

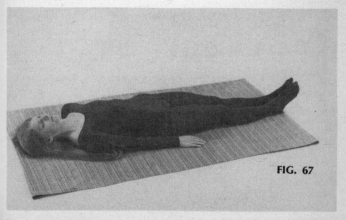

FIG. 67

14. PLOUGH (Halasana)

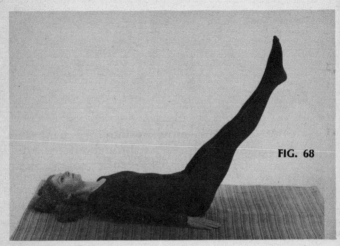

FIG. 68 — In a lying position lower your eyelids. *Inhale and retain.* Raise the legs and swing them back exactly as in the Shoulder Stand.

FIG. 69 — Lower the legs as far as possible and hold.

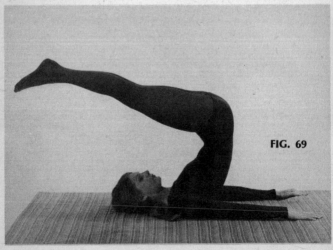

PHYSICAL EFFECTS: provides intensive concave stretching and strengthening throughout the entire back and spine; relieves tension; promotes flexibility.

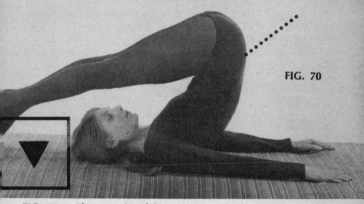

FIG. 70

FIG. 70 — The completed first position. The knees are straight, the feet as close in toward the head as possible.

Hold for twenty seconds. *Feel* the emphasis on the lower back and spine.

Visualize the root center at the base of the spine, the Muladhara chakra.

Exhale slowly and completely.

Without pause inhale and retain.

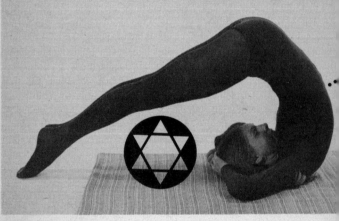

FIG. 71

FIG. 71 — *Retaining the air,* bring the arms up and clasp the hands on top of the head. Next inch the feet backward as far as possible. The knees remain straight. This is the second position.

Hold for twenty seconds. The emphasis has now shifted from the lower to the middle area of the back. *Feel* this area. Practice visualizing the heart center, the Anahata chakra.

Exhale slowly and completely.

Without pause inhale and retain.

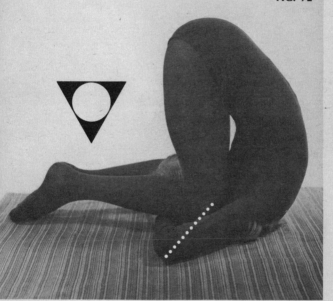

FIG. 72

FIG. 72 — Lower the knees to touch the floor within the arms. This is the third position.

Hold for twenty seconds. The pressure has now shifted from the middle back to the neck. *Feel* this area. Practice visualizing the throat center, the Vishuddha chakra.

Exhale slowly and breathe normally.

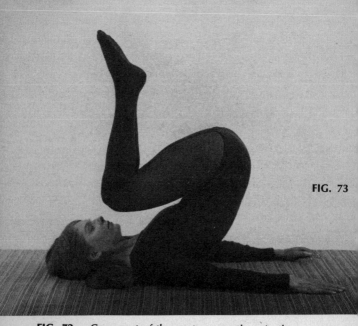

FIG. 73 — Come out of the posture exactly as in the Shoulder Stand.

Rest for approximately thirty seconds and hold the mind steady. Concentration on the breathing always prevents the mind from wandering.

Inhale and repeat.

Perform the three positions of the Plough twice.

15. BACK STRETCH (Paschimottanasana)

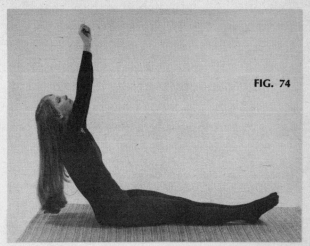

FIG. 74

FIG. 74 — In a seated position lower the eyelids and extend the legs, feet together.

Begin the inhalation. Slowly raise the arms to the indicated position. The trunk and head bend backward. *Complete the inhalation at this point.*

FIG. 75 — *Retain the air.* Bend forward slowly and hold the farthest part of the legs that you can reach without strain.

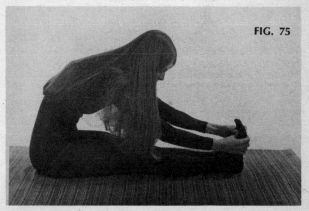

FIG. 75

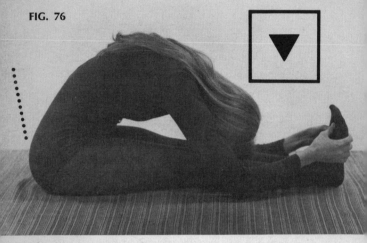

FIG. 76

FIG. 76 — Lower the head as far as possible toward the knees and hold. Fig 76 depicts the final position in which the hands hold the soles of the feet and sufficient flexibility has been developed to enable the elbows to touch the floor. Hold your extreme position (however elementary or advanced) for twenty seconds. Focus on the base of the spine and *feel* the stretching in that area. Practice visualizing the root center, the Muladhara chakra.

Begin the slow exhalation. Slowly straighten the trunk to the upright position and simultaneously draw the hands up the legs.

Complete the exhalation as the trunk becomes upright with the hands resting on the knees. Relax for several seconds, breathing normally and fixing the mind on the breathing.

Inhale and repeat.

Perform three times.

16. HEAD STAND (Viparitakarani)

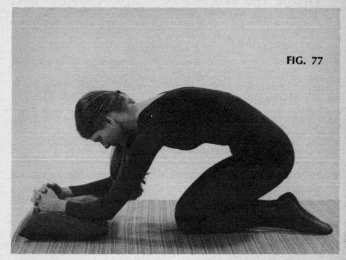

FIG. 77

FIG. 77 — Place a small pillow or folded mat beneath your head.

Interlace your fingers and lower your elbows and forearms to the floor so that they form a triangle. The eyes remain open.

FIG. 78 — Rest the top of your head on the mat; the back of your head is cradled firmly in your clasped hands.

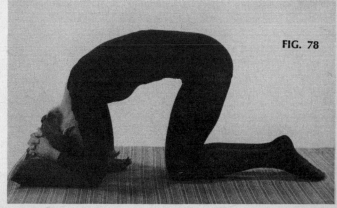

FIG. 78

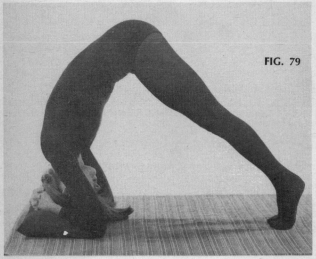

FIG. 79

FIG. 79 — Place your toes on the floor and push up so that your body forms an arch.

FIG. 80 — Walk forward on your toes and move your knees as close as possible to your chest.

PHYSICAL EFFECTS: promotes and aids in regulation of blood pressure and circulation; revitalizes the brain; helps to maintain alertness and prevent hardening of the arteries; promotes correct vision and hearing; improves the complexion and the condition of the scalp and hair.

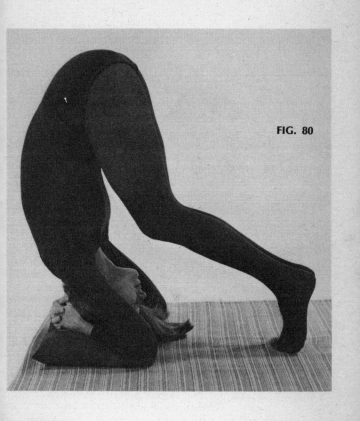

FIG. 80

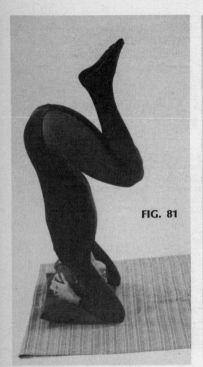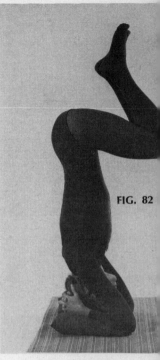

FIG. 81

FIG. 82

FIG. 81 — Push off the floor lightly with your toes and transfer your weight so that it is evenly distributed between your head and forearms. This is the Modified Head Stand and you should become secure in this position before attempting to straighten the legs. It may require some weeks of practice to master the modified position. After each attempt, simply return the feet to the floor and relax with the head down. Three attempts are sufficient in any one practice session.

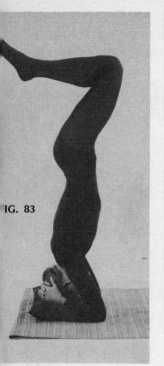

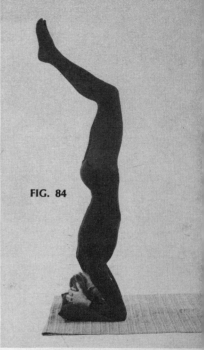

IG. 83

FIG. 84

FIG. 82; FIG. 83; FIG. 84 — Begin to straighten the legs slowly. You must become secure in moving into the final position very slowly. If you attempt to lurch into the completed posture you will never truly master the Head Stand.

If you become shaky at any point, return the feet to the floor. Rest and make another attempt.

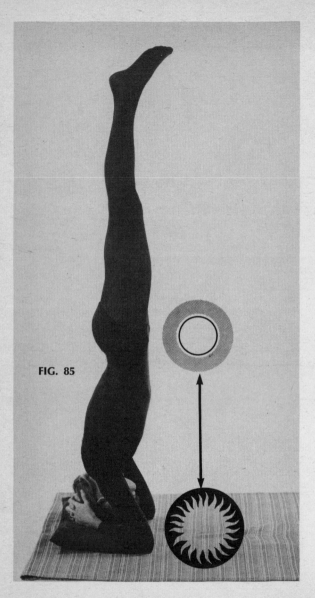

FIG. 85

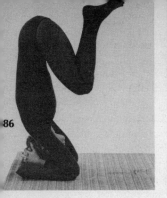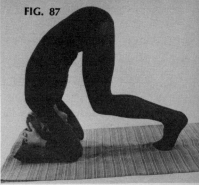

FIG. 85 — The completed posture. The body is as straight as possible, but can be relaxed. Many students find it necessary to keep their eyes open in order to maintain balance. Once secure in the completed position you can attempt lowering the eyelids to the three-quarter position. *There is no suspension of breath.* The breathing is regular and the physical point of concentration is on the breathing during the hold. Begin with ten seconds and very gradually work up to three minutes. Do not exceed three minutes until the posture has become *absolutely effortless* for you. Then you can continue to add time as comfortable. *Nothing forced and no strain imposed* is the ever-present principle that obtains in the practice of Hatha Yoga.

The visualization is unique in the Head Stand. Certain processes that ordinarily occur in the areas of the solar plexus and at the root of the palate and that are designated respectively as the "sun" and "moon" spheres are reversed in this inverted position. Our visualization reinforces the exchange of the sun and moon attributes. While in the inverted position we alternate continually between the visualization of the *moon in the navel area* and the *sun in the palate area*. First fix the moon in the navel area and hold the image for approximately fifteen seconds. Then move to the palate area and there fix a radiating sun for approximately fifteen seconds. Continue to alternate on this basis for the duration of the inversion. The Head Stand is a *mudra*.

FIG. 86; FIG. 87 — Come out of the posture with poise and balance. Lower your knees slowly to your chest and then lower your feet to the floor.

Remain with your head down for approximately one minute. When perfected, the Head Stand is performed only once.

187

17. DEEP RELAXATION (Savasana)

FIG. 88 — In a lying position lower the eyelids. Breathe normally. Beginning with the feet, direct your consciousness very slowly and very deliberately through each area of the body: the feet, calves, thighs, groin, buttocks, abdomen, chest, back; then down to the hands, arms, shoulders, neck, face, and head. As you become aware of each of these areas, attempt to *feel* it acutely and then to relax it in the extreme. Some areas may require several stages of "letting go" in order to achieve their ultimate relaxation. That is, relaxing one set of muscles you may find that there are others in the same area that are still contracted. Certain muscles may relax only partially and several attempts will be necessary to attain the ultimate state. Take as long as is required to place the entire body in the deep relaxation condition. Once this is accomplished the physical point of concentration is the slow, regular rhythm of the inhalations and exhalations.

The metaphysical practice is the visualization of the Sahasrara, the lotus of a thousand petals. Visualize a multitude of luminous, shimmering petals radiating from the crown of the head and encircling it. Maintain an almost blinding illumination. Reinforce the luminosity whenever it begins to fade. Continue the visualization until indications of fatigue are experienced. The duration can be gradually extended. This is a technique that imparts great revitalization to the entire organism.

**PHYSICAL EFFECTS: eliminates tension through-
out the organism and promotes restfulness and
quietude whenever necessary.**

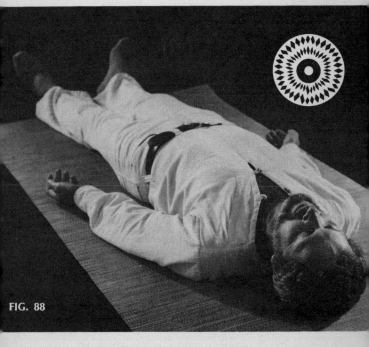

FIG. 88

The following three techniques (18, 19, and 20) are mudras and can be practiced only by those students who have mastered the Full-Lotus.

18. RAISED LOTUS (Maha Vedha)

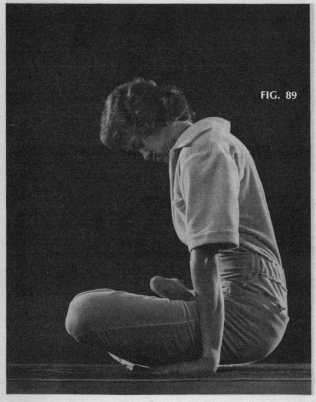

FIG. 89

FIG. 89 — Seated in Padmasana, *inhale and retain.*
Apply the bandhas as taught previously: tongue, chin, abdomen, anus. (See p. 128).
Place the hands as illustrated and raise the body slowly, steadily, and evenly several inches from the floor.

PHYSICAL EFFECTS: revitalizes; strengthens the arms; develops balance.

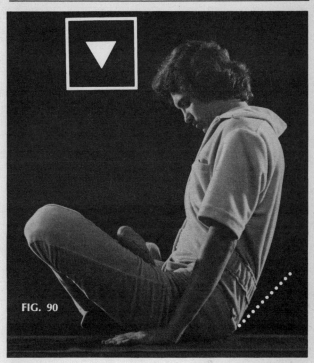

FIG. 90

FIG. 90 — Very cautiously and very gently lower the body with sufficient momentum to effect a slight jar at the base of the spine. It should be obvious that the greatest care must be exercised in lowering the body so that only a gentle impact is experienced between the base of the spine and the floor.

Direct the consciousness to the point of impact. Practice visualizing the Muladhara chakra.

Repeat once or twice more during this same retention.

Upon conclusion, raise the head, relax the bandhas, and *exhale.*

Rest a few moments and repeat, performing five to six lowerings in all.

19. LOCKED LOTUS
(Bandha Padmasana)

FIG. 91 — Seated in Padmasana, *exhale deeply and suspend breathing*. The lungs are now empty and remain empty.

Perform Uddiyana (the Abdominal *Lift*, not simply the Contraction) and the Anal Contraction.

Cross the arms behind the back with the left arm on top.

Hold the left big toe with the fingers of the left hand and the right big toe with the fingers of the right hand. At first it will probably be necessary to practice with only the fingers of the right hand holding the right toe, or vice versa— whichever is the easier. Gradually the necessary flexibility will be attained.

Work toward a thirty-second hold.

Direct the consciousness to the abdominal area. Visualize the Manipura chakra (the navel center).

Relax the Lift and the Contraction; release the toes. Return the arms to the knees. *Breathe normally*.

Perform only once.

PHYSICAL EFFECTS: promotes suppleness; tones the spine, develops good posture.

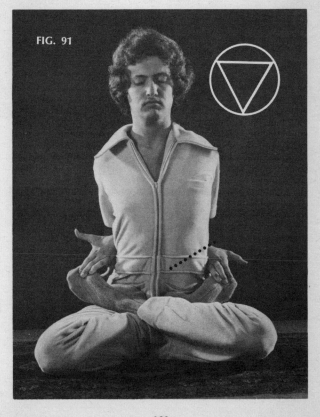

FIG. 91

20. YOGA MUDRA

FIG. 92 — Seated in Padmasana, clasp the hands behind the back.

Suspend breathing without any special inhalation or exhalation. That is, simply stop breathing (this is *kevala* kumbhaka).

Bend forward and touch the top of the head to the floor, as close in as possible. Breathing remains suspended.

Direct the consciousness to the point in the spine where the greatest emphasis is felt. Visualize a cross (formed by the position of the body).

Hold as long as possible. Work toward one minute. Breathing remains suspended throughout.

Straighten the trunk and *resume normal respiration*.

Perform only once.

Pranayama

There are at least ten breath-control exercises (kumbhakas) that are taught in the classical Hatha Yoga texts. For the student who is not devoting a very considerable part of his day to the practice of Hatha Yoga it is completely impractical to undertake the regular practice of such a large number of breathing techniques. And unless these *are* undertaken with precise regularity they cannot fulfill their objectives. Therefore, as a matter of practicality, we teach two essential breathing exercises that will accomplish the objectives of this course. These *can* be perfected and practiced regularly to great advantage by the student who is serious, but who is, nonetheless, limited in time.

The objectives of the following two exercises are:

1. To gain emotional stability and experience a general improvement in physical health.

2. To render the entire organism fit for concentration/meditation.

3. To cleanse the nadis in preparation for the esoteric practice of Hatha Yoga.

FIG. 92

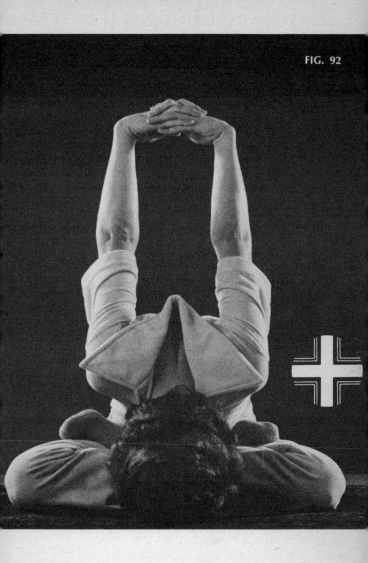

ABDOMINAL-CHEST QUICK
BREATHING (Kapalabhati, Bhastrika)

This is a breathing exercise, comprised of a series of short, quick, forceful movements, that is performed first with the abdomen and then with the chest.

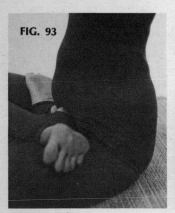
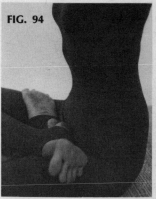

FIG. 93

FIG. 94

FIG. 93; FIG. 94 — Sit in one of the cross-legged postures. The Full-Lotus is the most desirable; if this is possible, make certain that the feet, heels, spine, and hands are in the proper positions. Either of the other two positions are satisfactory but the student should continue to practice for attainment of Padmasana.

Execute a short, quick inhalation through the nose and *simultaneously* expand the abdomen. This is the same movement that was learned in the Complete Breath, but now it is performed quickly.

Without pause execute a quick and forceful contraction of the abdomen so that the air is expelled through the nose in a short spurt and the lungs are emptied.

Without pause begin the next inhalation and the expansion of the abdomen.

The chest moves as little as possible; the breathing is almost silent. The movements are quick but must be done *rhythmically* and with precision.

Begin with ten repetitions, performing approximately one per second, and gradually increase to fifty, performing approximately three per second.

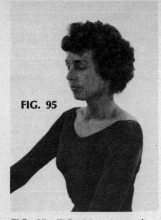

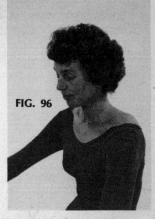

FIG. 95; FIG. 96 — Immediately upon completion of the abdominal movements transfer the breathing to the chest. That is, there is no pause between the last of the abdominal movements and the first of the chest movements. The chest expands during inhalation and contracts as the air is expelled. Movement in the abdomen is held to a minimum. This chest breathing will have to be performed somewhat slower than the abdominal breathing, and sound in the nostrils and throat will be more pronounced, but the pattern is the same: the chest is expanded as much as possible during a short, quick inhalation and, without pause, contracted quickly and forcefully to push the air completely from the lungs and out the nose.

The movements are, as with the abdominal breathing, continuous and *rhythmic*.

Begin with five movements, performing approximately one per second and gradually increase to twenty-five, performing approximately two per second.

The point of concentration in both the abdominal and chest breathing is only on the counting of the breaths.

Upon completion of the chest movements (that is, after the last exhalation), suspend all breathing for a few moments (the lungs are empty) and then perform a very deep Complete Breath. Retention of the air and application of the three bandhas are included. (Rather than the Half-Lotus, as suggested under directions for the "Complete Breath," this Complete Breath will be done in the Full-Lotus, providing, of course, it has been assumed for the abdominal-chest movements.)

197

PHYSICAL EFFECTS: cleanses and strengthens the respiratory system; increases lung capacity.

FIG. 97 — Following the exhalation of the Complete Breath, sit very quietly for a short time. Breathing will be naturally slowed. The point of physical concentration is in becoming aware of the extremely light, peaceful state of the entire organism. It is now "charged" in a manner that cannot be easily described. The metaphysical practice is the visualization of the triangle formed by the position of the body.

The concentration/visualization should consume approximately thirty seconds. This completes one round of Abdominal-Chest Quick Breathing:

Abdominal Breathing	10–50 repetitions
Chest Breathing	5–25 repetitions
Complete Breath	Once

Perform five rounds.

The advanced student, who has practiced seriously for a lengthy period of time and has become extremely proficient in this exercise, increases the repetitions. It is not unusual for such a student to perform one hundred or more Abdominal Breaths and follow them with fifty or more Chest Breaths for each round. In this case the respirations are extremely rapid and movement in the abdomen and chest is minimal.

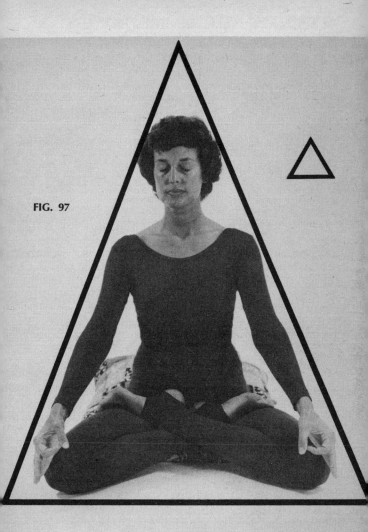

FIG. 97

ALTERNATE NOSTRIL BREATHING
(Chandra-Surya Kumbhaka)

The process of respiration brings prana into the subtle body through ida, a major nerve channel that is connected to the left nostril and is symbolically designated as the moon (chandra) channel, and through pingala, a nerve channel of equal importance that is connected to the right nostril and is symbolically designated as the sun (surya) channel.

The practice of Alternate Nostril Breathing—

1. Has a direct and immediate effect on the emotions and ordinary mind; both are dramatically stabilized and quieted.

2. Equalizes the quantity of prana that is introduced into the various central distribution points of the subtle body through ida and pingala.

3. Acts to cleanse these two principal nadis in preparation for the entrance of the prana into the sushumna.

PHYSICAL EFFECTS: as indicated above.

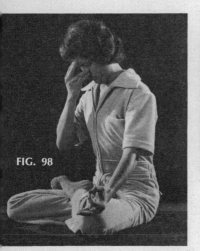

FIG. 98

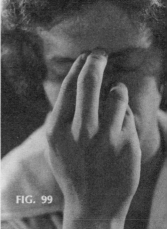

FIG. 99

FIG. 98; FIG. 99 — Again, the Full-Lotus is the traditional posture that is to be assumed but either of the other two will be satisfactory.

Rest the left hand in the indicated mudra on the left knee.

Study the illustrations. Place the tip of your right thumb lightly against the right nostril and the ring and little fingers lightly against the left. The index and middle fingers are together and they rest on the Ajna chakra with light pressure that is maintained throughout the exercise.

Exhale deeply, slowly, and quietly through both nostrils.

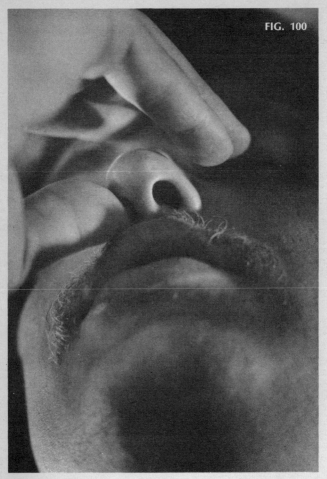

FIG. 100

FIG. 100 — Close the right nostril by pressing the thumb against it. Slowly and quietly inhale deeply through the left nostril. During this inhalation the body movements of the Complete Breath are executed in an extremely modified manner: the abdomen is only slightly expanded, and then the chest is only slightly expanded while the abdomen is slightly contracted. This inhalation is completed during a rhythmic count of eight.

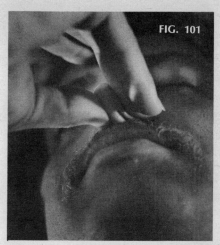

FIG. 101

FIG. 101; FIG. 102 — Keep the right nostril closed and now press the *left* closed so that both nostrils are closed. Maintain the pressure on the Ajna chakra. Retain the air during a rhythmic count of eight. As this count begins apply the bandhas: tongue, chin, abdomen, and anus.

FIG. 103 — Release the *right* nostril (the left remains closed). Exhale slowly, deeply, and quietly through the right nostril in a rhythmic count of eight. As this count begins, raise the head and relax all bandhas.

When the exhalation is completed do not pause but immediately begin the next inhalation through the *right* nostril (this is the same nostril through which you have just exhaled). Inhale a deep, quiet breath in a rhythmic count of eight. The left nostril remains closed.

Keep the left nostril closed and now press the *right* closed so that once again both are closed. Apply the *bandhas* as in Fig. 101. Retain the air during a rhythmic count of eight.

Raise the head and relax all bandhas.

Release the *left* nostril (the right remains closed) and exhale deeply and quietly in a rhythmic count of eight.

Now you have returned to the original starting point. Each time you return to this starting point you have completed one round of Alternate Nostril Breathing.

Without pause, keeping the right nostril closed, begin a deep, quiet inhalation through the *left* nostril.

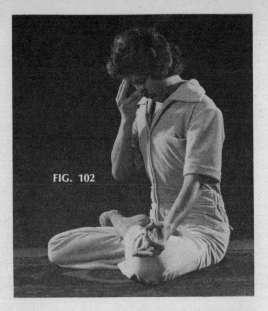

FIG. 102

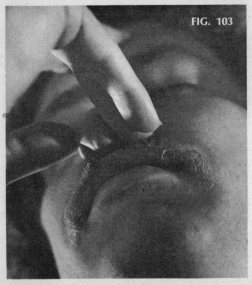

FIG. 103

Begin with four rounds and add one round each week until you reach seven rounds.

The count is of the utmost importance. The above directions, calling for a count of eight during inhalation, eight during retention, and eight during exhalation, are for the beginning stages of the exercise. (Remember that this counting is most smooth and rhythmic; there are no interruptions.) As proficiency is gained in breathing, counting, physical movements, and application of the bandhas the rhythm is changed. You must gradually work toward the rhythm that has a ratio of 1:4:2. In the actual counting this ratio is translated as four during inhalation, sixteen during retention, eight during exhalation. This is an advanced rhythm and requires serious practice to master because it must be constant and all movements smooth and coordinated

Summary:

Inhale through left	Count 8 or 4
Retain; both closed	Count 8 or 16
(apply bandhas)	
Exhale through right	Count 8 or 8
(release bandhas)	

Without pause:

Inhale through right	Count 8 or 4
Retain; both closed	Count 8 or 16
(apply bandhas)	
Exhale through right	Count 8 or 8
(release bandhas)	

This completes one round.
Begin the next round:

Inhale through left	Count 8 or 4
Etc.	

The attention is to be fully concentrated on the counting. At no time is the mind permitted to wander while the counting becomes "automatic."

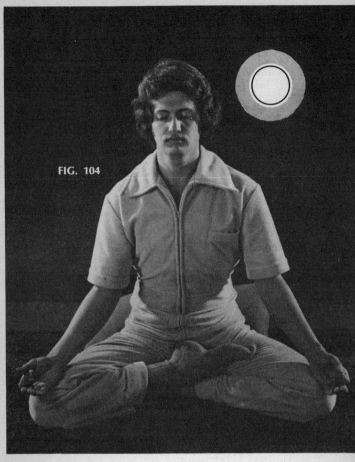

FIG. 104 — At the conclusion of the final round, sit very still for as long as is desired. If discomfort is being experienced because of extended sitting in the Full-Lotus, you may quietly change to the Half-Lotus. Breathing will be naturally slowed. Again, the point of physical concentration is in becoming aware of the extremely peaceful, elevated state of the entire organism. The metaphysical practice is the visualization of the Ajna chakra. Reinforce the image of this center whenever it begins to fade.

APPENDIX A

Practice Guide

This guide has been developed from the premise that the student is limited in time but will devote approximately forty-five minutes daily to serious practice. Imposing this time limitation necessitates dividing the techniques into two groups that are to be alternated on a daily basis: Monday—Group A; Tuesday—Group B; Wednesday—Group A; Thursday—Group B, etc.

Certain techniques are included in both Group A and Group B.

It is acceptable that the student divide either group into two segments and practice with the first segment earlier in the day and the second segment later in the day.

It is acceptable that, time permitting, the student perform Group A in its entirety earlier in the day and Group B in its entirety later in the day.

GROUP A	GROUP B
Kapalabhati-Bhastrika[1]	Kapalabhati-Bhastrika[1]
Complete Breath Standing	Complete Breath Standing
Rishi's Posture	Chest Expansion
Balance Posture	Triangle
Abdominal Lift	Abdominal Lift
Twist	Backward Bend
Cobra	Alternate Leg Stretch
Locust	Shoulder Stand
Bow	Plough
Head Stand	Back Stretch
Raised Lotus; Locked Lotus; Yoga Mudra[2]	Raised Lotus; Locked Lotus; Yoga Mudra[2]
Alternate Nostril Breathing	Deep Relaxation
Concentration/Meditation[3]	Concentration/Meditation[3]

[1] Assume the indicated folded-leg posture for Kapalabhati-Bhastrika, Alternate Nostril Breathing, and Concentration/Meditation. Remember to apply the bandhas as directed.

[2] When the Full-Lotus has been perfected, perform the Raised Lotus, Locked Lotus, and Yoga Mudra. It usually requires less than three minutes to perform all three.

[3] The preceding techniques of the practice session prepare the body and mind for serious Concentration/Meditation. The student may select his "seed" for concentration in accordance with the information presented in this book.

APPENDIX B

Application of Hatha Yoga to Physical and Emotional Problems

It has been our experience that various physical and emotional problems have frequently responded in a highly favorable manner to Hatha Yoga practice. The tables below indicate those techniques that can aid in achieving certain objectives or be applied to particular problems. These tables are not suggested as an alternative to medical treatment; rather, with the physician's approval, they offer the possibility of a dynamic form of physical therapy that can work to great advantage in conjunction with the general treatment that has been prescribed.

In electing to apply any of the indicated "problem" routines the student **must not neglect to perform the entire program of practice as presented in the "Practice Guide"** (unless directed otherwise by his physician). He should simply devote additional time to the indicated techniques, either by increasing the number of repetitions in the course of his regular practice or by performing **only** the "problem" routine at another time of the day.

(The numbers in the parentheses refer to the techniques, not the pages.)

ABDOMEN
(strengthened, firmed, raised)
Abdominal Lift (6)
Shoulder Stand (13)
Plough (14)
Locust (10)

ARMS
(including shoulders and hands; firmed, strengthened, developed)
Chest Expansion (2)
Locust (10)
Triangle (4)
Head Stand (16)

Raised Lotus (18)
Locked Lotus (19)

ARTHRITIS
The slow motion movements and "holds" of Hatha Yoga have provided dramatic relief for the arthritis victim. With his physician's approval, all of the less demanding asanas can be undertaken in an extremely modified manner by the patient. The movements can be

limited to a few inches and the "holds" maintained for only a few seconds each. It is gratifying to observe how quickly patients are able to extend these movements and holds. We contend that, at present, only this type of **self-manipulation** in conjunction with a Yoga-type diet holds the possibility of a natural cure for arthritis.

BACK
(all areas strengthened, firmed; stiffness and tension relieved)
Back Stretch (15)
Cobra (9)
Locust (10)
Bow (11)
Plough (14)
Twist (7)
Chest Expansion (2)
Rishi's Posture (3)

BALANCE
(development of equilibrium and poise)
Balance Posture (5)
Shoulder Stand (13)
Head Stand (16)
Rishi's Posture (3)
Backward Bend (8)

BLOOD
(circulation improved, pressure regulated)
Complete Breath
Chest Expansion (2)
Shoulder Stand (13)
Head Stand (16)
Cobra (9)
Locust (10)
Plough (14)

Yoga Mudra (20)
Alternate Nostril Breathing

BRAIN
(revitalized)
Identical with BLOOD

CHEST
(expanded, developed; bust developed)
Chest Expansion (2)
Cobra (9)
Bow (11)
Backward Bend (8)

CONSTIPATION
Abdominal Lift (6)

FACE
(complexion improved)
Identical with BLOOD

FEET
(including ankles and toes; strengthened, stiffness relieved)
Backward Bend (8)
Lotus Postures

HEADACHES
Alternate Nostril Breathing
Deep Relaxation (17)
Chest Expansion (2)
Cobra (9)
Shoulder Stand (13)
Head Stand (16)

LEGS
(thighs and calves firmed, strengthened, developed, tension relieved)
Alternate Leg Stretch (12)
Locust (10)
Bow (11)
Plough (14)
Backward Bend (8)
Shoulder Stand (13)

Triangle (4)
Rishi's Posture (3)
Balance Posture (5)

LUNGS
(cleansed, capacity increased)
Complete Breath
Abdominal-Chest Breaths
Alternate Nostril Breathing
All asanas in which prescribed breathing is included

NERVOUS SYSTEM
(general tension and insomnia relieved)
Complete Breath
Chest Expansion (2)
Cobra (9)
Twist (7)
Back Stretch (15)
Shoulder Stand (13)
Alternate Nostril Breathing
Deep Relaxation (17)

POSTURE
(improved)
Chest Expansion (2)
Backward Bend (8)
Locked Lotus (19)
Bow (11)

RESPIRATORY ILLNESSES

The entire Yoga program with emphasis on the serious but nonstrenuous practice of Pranayama, has proven effective. The Yoga diet is an essential part of this program.

SCALP-HAIR
Head Stand (16)

SPINE
(vertebrae strengthened and adjusted; stiffness and tension relieved)
Identical with BACK

WEIGHT CONTROL
(in conjunction with the Yoga diet)
Reduced in waist and hips:
Abdominal Lift (6)
Shoulder Stand (13)
Plough (14)
Triangle (4)
Twist (7)
Reduced in buttocks, thighs and calves:
Shoulder Stand (13)
Cobra (9)
Locust (10)
Bow (11)
Triangle (4)
Rishi's Posture (3)
Weight gain:
The entire Yoga program develops, firms and aids in proper assimilation of food and oxygen.

APPENDIX C

Yoga Nutrition

The major consideration of the Yogi in regard to nutrition and diet is the eating of small quantities of food that require a minimum expenditure of energy for digestion and that will leave the body light and satisfied while simultaneously providing proper nourishment and **maximum life force (prana).** These objectives are best achieved through foods that we term "natural"—that is, foods that can be ingested as close as possible to their original state. To the extent that foods are refined, canned, preserved, frozen, smoked, aged, colored, fumigated, enriched and otherwise processed they are **denatured;** they lose their prana and have an adverse effect for the practicing Yogi.

In the Western world the foods that are most desirable in the Yoga program are classified below. Related information follows the tables.

PROTEINS
Avocados
Legumes: beans, peas, lentils, soy beans and soy bean products
Nuts (unroasted and unsalted): almonds, cashews, pecans, walnuts, Brazil nuts
Coconuts (and coconut milk)
Mushrooms
Seeds: sunflower, pumpkin, etc.
See also **Dairy Foods**

Eliminate entirely or consume very sparingly
Meat, poultry, fish, Eggs

Eliminate entirely
All wafers, powders and tablets designated as "high protein" products

MINERALS
All edible fresh fruits and vegetables
(The only restrictions are individual preferences with respect to ease of digestion. Eliminate whatever is disagreeable.)

Consume as sparingly as possible
Frozen, bottled and canned fruits and vegetables.

GRAINS
All **whole** grain products. Breads, cereals, pastas, crackers, cakes, cookies, etc. that are made from

only whole grains will be so designated on their labels.

Eliminate entirely
All refined flour products. (Read the labels to determine the type of flour used in cereals, breads, cakes, etc. Do not be misled by the words "wheat" or "enriched." Only "whole grain" is satisfactory.)

DAIRY FOODS
(These are also fats and proteins)

Milk: certified raw, nonfat or low fat, goat, evaporated
Cheese: cottage (uncreamed), farmer, ricotta, Wisconsin cheddar
Yogurt (and all sour-milk products)
Butter (made from whole milk)

Eliminate entirely or consume very sparingly
Homogenized, pasteurized milk
Cream in all forms
Buttermilk
Sour Cream
All salted, spiced cheeses
Cream cheese
All yogurts that are flavored with fruits and syrups
Butter containing salt and animal fats (substitute vegetable margarines)

STARCHES
Brown rice
Bananas
Potatoes (baked, boiled)
Whole grain cereals, breads, crackers
Pumpkin
Barley
Rye

Eliminate entirely
White rice
Fried foods (potatoes, rice, etc.)
Refined flour products (including pies)
Corn starch products (puddings, etc.)

SUGARS
Fresh Fruits
Dried fruits: dates, figs, prunes, raisins, apricots, peaches, etc., all unsulphured
Molasses
Honey (uncooked, unbleached)
Raw Sugar
Beet Sugar
Cane Sugar (the cane stalks)
Carob (St. John's bread)

Eliminate entirely
All refined sugar products (read the labels)
All sugar substitutes designated as "low calorie" products

BEVERAGES
Water (pure; preferably without the chemicals added to the water supply of many municipalities)

All fresh fruit and vegetable juices

Vegetable broths and bouillons (without salt and chemicals)

Herb teas

Cereal beverages (as coffee substitutes)

Milk: low fat or non-fat, certified raw, goat

Eliminate entirely
Coffee
Tea
Milk (homogenized, pasteurized)
Alcoholic beverages
Colas and all syrup drinks (including "diet" colas)
Ice cream beverages

Consume sparingly
Bottled, frozen and canned juices

OILS
(Used for cooking and dressings; also classified as "fats")
Safflower oil
Sesame seed oil
Olive oil (pure)

CONDIMENTS
All edible herbs
Seasonings made from various combinations of vegetables and herbs

Eliminate entirely
Common salt (sodium chloride) and as many products containing such salt as possible
Catsup, mustard and all similar commercial products used to flavor "junk" foods

Consume sparingly
Vinegar
All "hot" spices such as ginger, peppers, etc.

Fruits and vegetables should be eaten raw, **including the skins,** whenever possible. Steaming, baking and broiling are the best cooking methods for our objectives. Avoid frying foods or using any substance that produces grease in cooking. Never boil or overcook foods, especially vegetables; heat them only until tenderized. Overcooking destroys prana. Vegetables should always retain crispness and never become soggy. Save and use as a broth or stock the juice produced from the cooking of vegetables. If one's digestion will not permit certain fruits being consumed in a raw state then they should be stewed or baked lightly. Honey, in moderation, may be added, but never sugar. Fresh fruits and vegetables are always our first choice. Frozen products are a second choice when fresh produce is unavailable. Bottled and canned fruits and vegetables, and fruit and vegetables juices rank very low on our list; almost all have sugar, salt, various condiments and chemicals added.

Dried fruits such as prunes, apricots and raisins are an excellent source of natural sugar energy and perfect for "snacks." If necessary they may be soaked for easier digestion. It is essential that all dried fruits **not have sulphur added.** (Unsulphured dried fruits are available in Health Food stores.)

Meat, poultry, fish, crustacea should be eliminated or consumed very sparingly. From a metaphysical standpoint, these foods lower the vibrations of the organism and produce restlessness. From a spiritual standpoint, the slaughter of millions upon millions of living creatures annually must be abhorred. From the physical standpoint, we contend that flesh foods place a stress on the digestive system and require more of an expenditure of prana than the meat itself produces. It is our belief that protein of a superior quality, without the heaviness and stress of meat, poultry and fish is obtained from those foods listed under "Proteins" in our tables. The flesh foods "debate" has been ongoing for many decades. The only way for the aspiring student to directly experience the dynamics that are involved is to eliminate these foods from his diet for a period of approximately 30 days. Natural proteins as listed in our table should be substituted. At the end of the 30 day period the student should return to his usual quantities of flesh consumption. The profound letdown and sluggishness that are generally experienced throughout the organism when the ingestion of flesh foods is resumed is usually adequate proof that their intake should be radically reduced or, preferably, discontinued. This is an experiment that is compulsory for the author's personal students.

We strongly discourage the use of pills, powders, wafers and all agents that act as appetite deterrents. Such agents cannot deceive the body for long and the consumer usually pays in health one way or another. We also believe that "high protein" diets set the body on a type of fire. In the long run they do not increase but rather deplete vitality. Those who undertake diets that include large quantities of meat, eggs, powders, wafers, etc. will find that they are restless, loggy and cannot properly practice meditation. For the same reasons we discourage the ingestion of coffee, tea, alcohol, refined sugar products and the chemical sugar "substitutes."

Beginning Yoga students should undertake a fresh fruit juice fast for one to two days each week. This is done to initiate a cleansing process and to experience the lightness and serenity that results when the digestive system is allowed to remain at relative rest for a short period. Advanced students often undertake a **complete** fast in which only water is taken for several consecutive days. We highly recommend a moderate fasting program to every serious Yoga student. Excellent progress in Hatha and Raja is usually experienced during a fasting period.

People vary widely in their reactions to different foods and combinations thereof. Again, our emphasis is on each student **becoming a law unto himself** and carefully observing the reactions of what he is eating on his own particular, unique organism. The discriminating student will understand this "uniqueness" principle and not be influenced by the hard and fast rules for dieting that appear wherever one turns.

When denatured foods are decreased or eliminated and natural foods are substituted the taste buds gradually lose their need for the various spices, seasoning and sweeteners that are the main attractions of the denatured foods. In this manner, without waging a constant battle, the student simply loses his desire for those foods that usually cause digestive problems, excess weight, various manifestations of ill-health and, in our view, many emotional and mental disturbances.

Health Food stores, some of which leave much to be desired in the way they are operated, are still the best source for obtaining many of the foods listed in our tables. With prudent and comparative shopping in these stores, the student will find the way to satisfy his basic requirements. Additionally, certain Health Food stores now stock fruits and vegetables that are termed "organic," i.e. produce that has not been fumigated with chemical sprays.

As with Yoga practice, we urge the student not to

divulge his experiments in natural food eating unless his particular situation requires that members of his family be taken into his confidence. A great amount of prana is lost in speaking about these things, even to one's closest friends. The student should remain silent until he has made significant progress. Then he can speak if he wishes.

Those who are under the care of a physician should consult him before adopting any part of this program.

BIBLIOGRAPHY

It is difficult to obtain English translations of the following seven works. Any such translation would be acceptable. Large public libraries and metaphysical bookstores are possible sources.

Yogacudamany Upanishad
Yogasikho Upanishad
Yoga-Kundali Upanishad
Rig Veda

Hatha Yoga Pradipika
Siva Samhita
Geranda Samhita

In addition to the primary works listed above any of the numerous Vedas or Upanishads will be of value to the serious student.

Bhagavad Gita—(any edition).

Osborne, Arthur, *Ramana Maharshi and the Path of Self-Knowledge,* Samuel Weiser, New York, 1970.

Patanjali, *Yoga Sutras (Aphorisms)*—(any edition).

Woodroffe, Sir John, *The Serpent Power,* Ganesh & Co., Madras, 1972.

Hittleman, Richard, *Introduction to Yoga,* Bantam Books, New York, 1969.

Hittleman, Richard, *Yoga Natural Foods Cookbook,* Bantam Books, 1970.

Hittleman, Richard, *Yoga For Personal Living,* Paperback Library, New York, 1972.

ABOUT THE AUTHOR

RICHARD LOWELL HITTLEMAN is the world's most widely read author on the subject of Yoga. Born in New York City and introduced to Yoga as a child by a Hindu employee of his parents, Mr. Hittleman became fascinated with the subject and continued its practice throughout his school years. After receiving his Masters Degree from Columbia University he embarked upon extensive travel for the purpose of studying Yoga and related oriental disciplines. Mr. Hittleman began instructing Yoga in the early 1950s. His **Yoga for Health** programs, televised continuously since 1961, are seen throughout the United States and in many foreign countries. He is the author of ten books; his writings have appeared in various medical, dental and health journals and his instructional albums and tapes are utilized by more students than any Yoga material ever recorded. Mr. Hittleman lives with his family on the coast of Northern California where he conducts periodic workshops and teachers seminars.